○ Collins *gem*

Calorie
Counter

D0610915

This book has been compiled with the assistance
of hundreds of brand-name manufacturers.
Other sources are listed on page 65.

HarperCollins Publishers
77–85 Fulham Palace Road
Hammersmith W6 8JB

www.collins.co.uk

First published 1984
Ninth edition published 2009

ISBN 978-0-00-731762-2

Printed and bound in China
by Leo Paper Products Ltd.

Contents

Preface

The Collins Gem Calorie Counter is one of the most successful guides available for weight-watchers. In this new edition, you'll find a new selection of foods, reflecting the range of foods now available. *The Calorie Counter* doesn't just list the calorie content of each food; it gives its nutritional composition as well, and we have also updated this data. Calorie content is given in either 100g measurements, or per item where it seems logical to do so; an emphasis has been placed on providing the most accurate information in the most user-friendly format.

The book contains:

An introduction that explains about weight loss, the targets you may need to set and information on a healthy, calorie-controlled diet.

A listing of around 6,000 foods, including both everyday ingredients and many of the thousands of branded foods available in shops today.

Study the Contents pages (pages 3–9) and the Index to help identify the foods you are looking for. For each entry we give information on the following: calories, protein, carbohydrates and fat.

A selection of delicious recipes – all of which can form part of a calorie-controlled diet – demonstrating that counting calories is perfectly compatible with eating well.

It has long been known that the healthiest and most effective way to lose weight and maintain that loss is to combine a healthy, calorie-controlled diet with exercise. We hope that this guide will help you to plan the best way to restrict your calorie intake.

Useful Websites

www.bbc.co.uk/health/healthy_living/your _weight/ (excellent site with medical advice, tips, eating well, fitness and useful contacts)

www.nhs.uk/livewell/loseweight (excellent basic advice including tips and encouraging 'real stories')

www.eatwell.gov.uk (useful, practical information on healthy diet issues and on matters such as food labelling)

www.netdoctor.co.uk/health_advice/facts/ loseweight.htm (practical general site with plan outlines)

www.bdaweightwise.com (excellent site run by British Dietetic Association; can put you in touch with a dietitian) www.nutrition.org.uk (good, sensible advice based on research; can put you in touch with a nutritionist)

www.weightconcern.com (addresses physical and psychological needs of overweight people)

www.weightlossresources.co.uk (a wide range of information)

www.caloriecounter.co.uk (a general guide including useful special topics)

www.ibodz.com (exercise site with advice on exercise and weight loss)

www.recipezaar.com (US site with calorie-counted recipes from around the world)

Introduction

Calorie-counting has sometimes had a bad press, dismissed as being out of date and boring. Some diets have even gone so far as to announce that 'calories don't count'.

One of the reasons for the poor reputation of old-fashioned calorie counting is that there was an emphasis on obsessive calculating, on using low-calorie processed food and ready meals, and on sticking to the assigned calorie limits no matter what. This combination of factors made calorie counting almost impossible to stick to and proved to be impractical in the long term. There was no emphasis on enjoying a healthy diet – you could eat your allocated calories in chocolate if you wished – and an almost complete lack of flexibility. Other, newer, apparently more user-friendly ways of losing weight seemed much more interesting but, in the long term, most of these have proved to be every bit as unsustainable.

Calories, however, always do count. They are just a measure of energy. Take in more calories than your body uses and the weight goes on as the excess is stored as fat; use more calories than you take in and the weight comes off as the body uses the energy it has stored. Reducing calorie intake is how all effective diets work, and there's no magic solution that involves anything else.

To make sure that you can reduce your calorie intake reasonably accurately, you will have to count the calories in the food you eat and the liquids you drink. That doesn't have to be depressing; nor does it mean that you will have to walk around for the rest of your life with a notebook under your arm, this book in one hand and a calculator in the other. Successful dieters become 'calorie aware', able to spot the low-calorie, nutritionally sound option at a glance, and also have a mental library of quick calorie shortcuts (you'll find some at the end of this Introduction). Small changes can make a significant difference; for instance, weaning yourself off three cappuccinos a day and swapping to black coffee instead could save hundreds of calories. This book will help you to learn the values for all your favourites and serve as a quick reference in which to look up new foods. But successful calorie counting isn't just about adding up the figures and keeping them to a certain limit; it's about being healthy as well. Then it really can be the start of a process of sustainable change.

What's a calorie?

Calories are a simple measurement of available energy: not fat, just energy. When food is metabolised it produces heat, and that energy is measured in kilocalories (kCal). A single scientific calorie is a very small measurement of energy, and scientists use the 1000-calorie measure – the kilocalorie – instead. Outside scientific circles, kilocalories have become known as calories and in this book, as in most other contexts, 'calorie' is used instead of 'kilocalorie'.

All food contains calories and all calories are the same regardless of their origin, apart from exceptional circumstances. The real difference comes in the nutritional benefits food has and not in the calories it contains; energy is not the body's only requirement, which is why a healthy diet is critical. Like all living things, the human body requires chemical building blocks, the nutrients which enable it to grow, develop normally, maintain itself, repair damage, manufacture hormones and perform many other functions. An apple and a boiled sweet may well make the same number of calories of energy available to the body – about 50 – but they won't bring the same health benefits. Calorie counting does bring freedom as you are not tied to any particular diet plan, but freedom brings responsibility and you need to ensure that you are as healthy as possible.

Fad diets

Diets suggesting you omit an entire category of food, eat a lot of any particular food or any alleged 'miracle food' should ring alarm bells. So should any diets that promise rapid weight loss or that don't advise you to increase exercise – especially in the maintenance phase – as well as cut your food intake.

Assessing weight

It's important to be realistic when looking at what you want to weigh and at how long it will take to get there, and the first thing to do is gather some information. Measure your height and weight before you start but do so in metric units – metres and kilograms – as this makes assumptions less likely.

WAIST MEASUREMENTS

Check this first. Doctors take waist measurements seriously because people who carry excess fat round the waist are in the highest-risk category for high blood pressure, heart disease and strokes. If your waist measurement rises above 94cm (for men) and 80cm (for women) you are putting your health at risk. If it's above 102cm for men and above 88cm for women, your health is at serious risk and you should start a weight-loss programme as soon as possible. A related risk indicator is the waist-to-hip ratio. The waist is measured at the narrowest point and that figure is divided by the hip measurement at the widest point.

A high figure is more than 1.0 in men and 0.85 in women; a healthy value is anything below these.

THE BMI – BODY MASS INDEX

The most common place to begin a more detailed assessment is likely to be the BMI or Body Mass Index, which doctors and health professionals often use to calculate whether you are over- or underweight; it's a height to weight formula. There is a BMI table on pages 20–21, but if you want to get a more precise figure, or if you fall outside the range of the table, you can calculate it yourself. Divide your weight in kilograms by the square of your height in metres, i.e., weight ÷ height x 2.

For example, if you are 1.70m tall and weigh 68kg, then 1.70 x 1.70 = 2.89, and 68 ÷ 2.89 = 23.52. That's your BMI.

Find your height in metres and your weight in kilograms, and trace a line from each. Your BMI figure is where the two lines intersect.

Kg	m 1.52	1.54	1.56	1.58	1.60	1.62	1.64	1.66	1.68
46	19.9	19.4	19	18.4	18	17.5	17.1	16.7	16.3
48	20.8	20.2	19.7	19.2	18.7	18.3	17.8	17.4	17
50	21.6	21.1	20.6	20	19.5	19.1	18.6	18.1	17.7
52	22.5	21.9	21.4	20.8	20.3	19.8	19.3	18.8	18.4
54	23.3	22.8	22.2	21.6	21.1	20.6	20.1	19.6	19.1
56	24.2	23.6	23	22.4	21.9	21.4	20.8	20.3	19.9
58	25.1	24.5	23.9	23.2	22.7	22.1	21.6	21	20.6
60	26	25.3	24.7	24	23.4	22.9	22.3	21.7	21.3
62	26.8	26.2	25.5	24.8	24.2	23.7	23	22.4	22
64	27.7	27	26.3	25.6	25	24.4	23.8	23.2	22.7
66	28.6	27.8	27.2	26.4	25.8	25.2	24.5	23.9	23.4
68	29.4	28.7	28	27.2	26.6	26	25.3	24.6	24.1
70	30.3	29.5	28.8	28	27.3	26.7	26	25.4	24.8
72	31.1	30.4	29.6	28.8	28.1	27.5	26.8	26.1	25.5
74	32	31.2	30.4	29.6	28.9	28.2	27.5	26.8	26.2
76	32.9	32	31.3	30.4	29.7	29	28.2	27.5	27
78	33.8	32.9	32.1	31.2	30.5	29.8	29	28.3	27.7
80	34.6	33.8	32.9	32	31.2	30.5	29.7	29	28.4
82	35.5	34.6	33.7	32.8	32	31.3	30.5	29.7	29.1
84	36.3	35.4	34.6	33.6	32.8	32.1	31.2	30.4	29.8
86	37.2	36.3	35.4	34.4	33.6	32.8	32	31.1	30.5
88	38.1	37.2	36.2	35.2	34.4	33.6	32.8	31.9	31.2
90	39	38	37	36	35.1	34.3	33.5	32.6	31.9
92	39.9	38.8	37.9	36.8	35.9	35.1	34.2	33.3	32.6
94	40.7	39.7	38.7	37.6	36.7	35.9	34.9	34	33.3
96	41.5	40.5	39.5	38.4	37.5	36.6	35.7	34.8	34
98	42.4	41.3	40.3	39.2	38.3	37.4	36.4	35.5	34.7
100	43.3	42.2	41.1	40	39.1	38.2	37.2	36.2	35.5
102	44.1	43	42	40.8	39.8	38.9	37.9	37	36.2
104	45	43.9	42.8	41.6	40.6	39.7	38.7	37.7	36.9
106	45.9	44.7	43.6	42.4	41.4	40.4	39.4	38.4	37.6
108	46.7	45.5	44.4	43.2	42.2	41.2	40.1	39.1	38.3

1.70	1.72	1.74	1.76	1.78	1.80	1.82	1.84	1.86	1.88	1.90
15.9	15.5	15.1	14.8	14.5	14.2	13.9	13.5	13.3	13	12.7
16.6	16.2	15.8	15.5	15.1	14.8	14.5	14.1	13.8	13.6	13.3
17.3	16.9	16.5	16.1	15.8	15.4	15.1	14.7	14.4	14.1	13.8
18	17.6	17.1	16.8	16.4	16	15.7	15.3	15	14.7	14.4
18.7	18.2	17.8	17.4	17	16.6	16.3	15.9	15.6	15.3	14.9
19.4	18.9	18.5	18.1	17.7	17.3	16.9	16.5	16.2	15.9	15.5
20.1	19.6	19.1	18.7	18.3	17.9	17.5	17.1	16.7	16.4	16.1
20.8	20.3	19.8	19.4	18.9	18.5	18.1	17.7	17.3	17	16.6
21.5	20.9	20.5	20	19.5	19.1	18.7	18.3	17.9	17.5	17.1
22.1	21.6	21.1	20.6	20.2	19.7	19.3	18.9	18.5	18.1	17.7
22.8	22.3	21.8	21.3	20.8	20.4	19.9	19.4	19.1	18.7	18.3
23.5	22.9	22.4	21.9	21.4	21	20.5	20	19.7	19.2	18.8
24.2	23.6	23.1	22.6	22.1	21.6	21.1	20.6	20.2	19.8	19.4
24.9	24.3	23.8	23.2	22.7	22.2	21.7	21.2	20.8	20.4	19.9
25.6	25	24.4	23.9	23.3	22.8	22.3	21.8	21.4	21	20.5
26.3	25.7	25.1	24.5	24	23.5	23	22.4	22	21.5	21
27	26.4	25.7	25.1	24.6	24	23.6	23	22.5	22.1	21.6
27.7	27	26.4	25.8	25.2	24.7	24.2	23.6	23.1	22.7	22.1
28.4	27.7	27.1	26.4	25.9	25.3	24.8	24.2	23.7	23.2	22.7
29.1	28.4	27.7	27.1	26.5	25.9	25.4	24.8	24.3	23.8	23.2
29.8	29.1	28.4	27.7	27.1	26.5	26	25.3	24.8	24.4	23.8
30.4	29.7	29	28.4	27.8	27.1	26.6	25.9	25.4	24.9	24.4
31.1	30.4	29.7	29	28.4	27.8	27.2	26.5	26	25.5	24.9
31.8	31.1	30.4	29.7	29	28.4	27.8	27.1	26.6	26.1	25.5
32.5	31.8	31	30.3	29.6	29	28.4	27.7	27.2	26.6	26
33.2	32.4	31.7	31	30.3	29.6	29	28.3	27.7	27.2	26.6
33.9	33.1	32.3	31.6	30.9	30.2	29.6	28.9	28.3	27.8	27.1
34.6	33.8	33	32.2	31.5	30.9	30.2	29.5	28.9	28.3	27.7
35.3	34.5	33.7	32.9	32.2	31.5	30.8	30.1	29.5	28.9	28.2
36	35.1	34.3	33.5	32.8	32.1	31.4	30.7	30	29.5	28.8
36.7	35.8	35	34.2	33.4	32.7	32	31.2	30.6	30	29.4
37.4	36.5	35.6	34.9	34	33.3	32.6	31.8	31.2	30.6	29.9

Now that you have your BMI figure, you can apply the BMI scale:

less than 15:	emaciated
15–18.9:	underweight
19–24.9:	average/healthy
25–29.9:	overweight
30 plus:	obese

If your BMI is in the emaciated or obese range, you should visit your doctor for advice as you could be seriously endangering your health. There are different BMI scales for children and adolescents, and some ethnic groups have different BMI ratings – for example, the WHO states that a BMI of 27.5 for someone of Asian origin carries the same health risks as a BMI of 30 for a Caucasian.

The BMI is a useful tool, although it doesn't give any indication of where fat is stored, which will affect the health risks you face – if your BMI is in the healthy band but your waist measurement is not, your health is still potentially at risk. There are also several groups for whom the formula doesn't apply. Pregnant women or heavily muscled athletes could appear overweight on the BMI scale; it doesn't allow for muscle mass. Nor does it differentiate by sex or build, but, as a broad generalisation, women and those of a slighter build should ideally be at the lower end of the healthy band, while men and those who have a larger frame should be towards the top.

Children
Children go through growth spurts, so if you are concerned about your child's weight talk to your GP first. Improving activity levels is a better place to start than counting a child's precise calorie intake, but you could begin by restricting obviously unhealthy items such as fizzy drinks, fatty snacks and sweets.

Setting a target
You can also use the BMI to give yourself a realistic target. Ideally, you want to be in the healthy band, with a BMI between 19 and 24.9. Here's an example of how it works in practice. If you are 1.64m tall and weigh 78kg, your BMI

is 29. To fall into the healthy band, you would need to weigh between 52 and 66kg. That's quite a drop, even at the minimum 12kg, let alone the 26kg it would take to get down to 52kg. A realistic weight-loss target is between 5 and 10 per cent of your starting body weight over six months to a year. Any more than that, any quicker than that, and you will struggle to keep the lost weight off in the long term and may damage your health on the way. In this case, losing 10 per cent would mean getting to about 70 kilograms – a more sensible aim, and close to the healthy BMI band. On achieving that, the next step would be to stop and stay at 70kg for a while before gently trying to lose some more.

When it comes to more precise timing, you should not try and lose more than 0.5kg a week; anything else is unsustainable and trying to lose weight more quickly than this is counter-productive. You do need to bear in mind that not all weeks are the same, either, and that losing anything on some weeks – holidays, for example – might be almost impossible. If that is the case, aim for staying the same; try not to put weight on!

Warning

Anyone who is considering trying to lose a lot of weight should consult their doctor first. You should also see your doctor before starting a diet if you have been overweight for years, have any long-term health problems or take medication for chronic conditions such as diabetes, angina, epilepsy or osteoporosis. It's especially important to check with your doctor if you have not done much exercise and are considering doing more. Make sure you are up to it, and don't be over-ambitious.

How many calories?

Given that there's an apparently simple principle at work – take in more calories than your body uses and the weight goes on; use more calories than you take in and the weight comes off – you might think that calculating a precise calorie intake figure for weight loss would be easy. Unfortunately, that's not the case. Human bodies are not machines and they do not work like them; there are too many variables.

It's possible to come up with a basic general guideline, however. Ideally, you need to eat between 500 and 600 calories less a day than your body uses in order to lose 0.5kg a week. Most women will lose that amount on 1,500 calories a day, most men on 1,900. It's dangerous to drop much below these figures, except under medical supervision. Spread the calories throughout the day – for example, on 1,500 calories, allow 300 for breakfast, 400 for lunch and 550 for dinner, with the remaining 250 for snacks, drinks including milk in tea or coffee, etc. Stick to three meals and two (healthy) snacks per day; it is very important not to skip meals or allow yourself to get hungry.

If you keep dieting and exercising without achieving your target, it may be that you are being unrealistic and trying to reach a weight that is unhealthy for you, so go back and check your targets again (check your intake, too, by keeping an accurate food diary – see pages 28–29 – including measuring and as few estimates as possible; portion sizes have a tendency to creep upwards).

Don't be tempted into trying crash diets, which often take calories below safe levels and promise to help you lose weight in a short period of time. They can pose a serious risk to health:

Your metabolism will slow down as your body tries to protect itself by hanging onto its fat stores and dropping its RMR (see pages 30–1), making it more difficult to shed weight. Once you stop actually dieting you are likely to pile the weight back on as your body is now using less energy – only you put on more than before. This leads to another crash diet, another gain in weight, and the overall effect is of weight gain over time rather than weight loss. Yo-yo dieting like this can have a significant impact on the heart.

Deprivation dieting or skipping meals can cause a drop in blood sugar levels, which leads to sugar cravings and an urge to binge, and upsets the delicate insulin balance (see pages 36–8). It also has an effect on the brain, which means that you will crave high-energy (and therefore high-calorie) food to compensate. Your body will use muscle tissue for energy rather than fat. Muscle tissue uses more calories than fat tissue, so your rate of weight loss is likely to slow down.

The more extreme the diet, the greater the likelihood that you will not be able to stick to it, leading to a cycle of self-recrimination, trying another diet and failing again.

Calorie counting in practice

Keeping a daily food diary is one of the most useful things you can do when you are dieting (you could do this on paper, using the templates at the back of the book, or electronically, whichever you prefer).People who keep an accurate record are more likely to be successful. This may be because seeing the food and calories in black and white has a salutary effect or because the process of making a note helps people stop and think.

Note down everything you eat as soon as you can; don't try to remember later what you have eaten, as you will inevitably forget some items and make mistakes about portion size. Most people do forget things, so be aware of that and try to ensure that you don't; the things you omit could make a big difference (some studies have shown under-recording by as much as 60 per cent, with the main omissions being drinks, snacks and healthy food!).

Do some rough mental planning in advance so that you don't run out of calories by midday, and remember that you need to eat three meals and two snacks – do not be tempted into skipping meals, especially breakfast. Where possible, weigh; buy yourself a set of spoon measures to use when cooking, and some slimmer's scales that weigh smaller quantities more clearly. If weighing is not possible, try and estimate, but note that this is what you have done. Recording will soon become second nature, and noting estimates will allow you to assess where things may have gone adrift if you have problems. Working out your subtotals as you go along will allow you to see whether you can afford that glass of wine or slice of cake in the evening or not. Tot up your calories at the end of the day.

Weighing yourself is not the only way of monitoring weight loss, and can even be confidence-destroying; there will be times when you have put on a little despite your best efforts, and others when your weight doesn't seem to shift at all. Changing measurements are another way, so take some starting measures – waist, hips, chest – and note them down. Or take a garment that is tight at the start of your diet, and assess how the fit improves as you lose weight.

If you do weigh yourself, like most people, do it only once a week at most; weight fluctuates perfectly normally from day to day and you want to look at an underlying trend. Make sure the scales are always in the same place and on a flat surface, weigh yourself at the same time of day – preferably first thing in the morning – and wearing roughly the same clothes. Do not become disheartened if there is some fluctuation from one week to the next, but if the overall tendency is upwards or your weight stalls for some time, you will need to check your calorie intake carefully and make sure you are not eating more (or even less, which can be equally bad in terms of stalls) than you should. Try taking a little more exercise, too.

Calories out – using energy

The human body uses the energy taken in three main ways. The most important of these is your Resting Metabolic Rate (RMR), which accounts for between 65 and 75 per cent of all the energy burned. This is the amount of energy your body expends while at rest on processes such as the circulation of the blood, keeping the heart beating, breathing, the production and release of hormones, and maintaining body temperature. RMR varies from person to person, partly because muscle burns more energy than fat, even when you're not moving. A kilogram of muscle can burn more than 120 kilocalories a day at rest, while a kilogram of fat burns 20 kCal or less. So the more muscle you have, the higher your RMR is likely to be, and the more energy you will burn without trying. This is one of the reasons why exercise is important, and particularly so when you are trying to maintain your new weight: it builds muscle.

The second way to burn energy is known as the Thermic Effect of Food, and it represents the amount of energy required to digest food. It's generally around 10 per cent of the calories eaten, but is negligible in practice when it comes to the whole picture.

The third way to burn energy is called the Thermic Effect of Exercise. It's the most variable percentage; athletes can burn a lot of energy in this way, but most people do not. The figures for energy expenditure during exercise depend on lots of different factors, such as muscle mass and the intensity of the effort put in; it's difficult to be objective. While it's possible to find figures online for different activities, they are subject to many qualifications (the simpler they appear, the less reliable they are – only use them as a general guideline). Even so, they may seem surprisingly low: a 65kg woman would only use 255 calories in half an hour's jogging, for example, though there would be some longer-term positive effects as well. One thing to note: exercising can make you hungrier, so watch that your food intake doesn't go up.

The most effective way to burn more calories is to raise your RMR by developing a more active lifestyle and forming more muscle, while eating less and eating more healthily. In modern Western societies, most people are more sedentary than they were in previous generations; we walk much less than our grandparents did, and our jobs often involve sitting down or being comparatively still for long periods. Improving on this can make a difference. It's important to remember that exercise doesn't just consist of playing team sports or working out, and that it has other benefits for your health.

There are official guidelines – in the UK, the recommendation is for 30 minutes of moderate exercise, five days a week, every week. 'Moderate' exercise should leave you feeling slightly breathless, so it means a brisk walk rather than a leisurely amble. Doubling the time wouldn't do any harm (60 minutes is recommended by some organisations), and it can be split up into smaller chunks throughout the day; in fact, research suggests this to be more effective. Incorporate more activity into your life. Walk or cycle to work, always take the stairs rather than a lift or escalator, and do some energetic gardening, housework or take the dog for a run when you get home. You could easily make up the 60 minutes total time without setting foot in a gym.

It's often said that overweight people have a 'slow metabolism'. In fact their RMR is often normal or higher, as it simply takes more energy to keep a larger body ticking over. As weight comes off, RMR will inevitably drop as the body requires less energy, but boosting muscle mass – muscle uses more energy – can help to counteract this effect. Your RMR will also decrease if you cut calories too dramatically; the body cannot distinguish between deliberate action on your part and a famine situation, and reacts by protecting itself and hanging on to its fat reserves – something that happens in crash diets. It will also decrease as you get older, by roughly 2 per cent for each decade over the age of 20, unless you take positive steps to keep it high. There's also a genetic element. Note that some diets and supplements may claim to 'increase your metabolic rate': treat these with scepticism.

It's almost impossible to produce a simple mathematical summary of how much energy you use along the lines of 'I will use a total of X calories today by doing A, B and C, so that's what I can eat.' There are online calculators which aim to give an objective figure, but they depend on potentially vague and subjective information, such as your assessment of how sedentary you are. The basic advice of 'eat less and do more' is just as valid as it ever was.

Calories in – food and drink

Calorie counting has to be matched with a healthy diet for long-term success; that's the only way to achieve the lifestyle change necessary for sustainable weight loss. There are two changes that will have an immediate impact. First, eat less processed food and fewer ready meals; second, cook more. When you cook, you control what you eat and how it's been prepared – and it doesn't have to take ages.

No single food contains all the nutrients the body needs, but a balanced and healthy diet does. A good balance of a wide variety of foods will ensure an adequate supply of nutrients, and that means striking a balance between the major food groups: carbohydrates, proteins and fats. The other substances that are necessary – micronutrients such as vitamins, minerals and phytochemicals as well as dietary fibre – come with a varied and healthy diet, one that is likely to contain a large variety of different foods. A healthy diet is particularly important if you are reducing the overall quantity of food you eat, as there's less slack to make up the difference.

CARBOHYDRATES

Carbohydrates are the body's main source of energy. They are found in plant-based foods – fruits, vegetables, grains and pulses – but are also present in others; cows' milk, for example, has more carbohydrate than either protein or fat. During digestion carbs are broken down into simple sugars such as glucose and released into the bloodstream. Insulin, a hormone that most people associate with diabetes, then helps the glucose enter the body's cells where it's used. The energy that comes from glucose provides most of the body's requirements, and any that is not needed is stored; some of this is converted into fat. Carbohydrates also help to regulate blood pressure, lower cholesterol levels and process fat, build amino acids, help the body absorb calcium and do many other things. Despite the assertions of the more extreme no-carb diets, there is no need to avoid them (even if it was possible). They form the basis of a healthy diet.

It is important, though, to choose wisely because not all carbs have the same impact. Some can help with weight loss while others definitely will not, and distinguishing between them is the basis of the GI (Glycaemic Index) diets. These enjoyed a wave of popularity not unlike that of the Atkins diet, but the GI diets were welcomed by medics where Atkins generally was not. This was because GI diets encouraged healthy eating and emphasised the best sort of carbohydrates – those with a low GI or glycaemic index. Portion control, however, was often a problem, and too many calories of healthy food are still too many calories.

The glycaemic index is a measure of the speed at which foods are broken down into the glucose that the body uses for energy, and is usually expressed as high, medium or low rather than as a precise figure. High GI foods are broken down very quickly and cause an almost immediate rise in blood sugar. Low GI foods are broken down much more slowly, keeping blood sugar levels steady. Any sharp rise in blood sugar is followed by an equally sharp drop, which sends a signal to the body that it needs more glucose to make up the difference – and the net result is feeling hungry shortly after eating something, which causes a spike. But that isn't the only impact. Insulin helps glucose enter the cells. Having high blood sugar levels means having high levels of insulin circulating in the blood, and insulin also inhibits the release of stored fat. Having high levels of insulin is no help when you are trying to lose weight, but it can also have a more serious impact on overall health. It's important to keep blood sugar levels as steady as possible, and choosing low GI foods can help.

FIBRE

Dietary fibre is a form of carbohydrate and is an essential part of the diet, although it doesn't provide any nutrients as such. There are two types of fibre: soluble and insoluble. Soluble fibre, such as that found in oats and apples, slows down the absorption of other carbs; insoluble fibre helps the digestion by adding bulk and absorbing water. Certain kinds of dietary fibre, such as oat bran, appear to lower levels of cholesterol in the blood, and fibre also contributes to the feeling of satisfaction after a meal. In general, high-fibre diets help to prevent type 2 diabetes and have been linked to lower rates of colon cancer. Most people eat too little fibre, but don't increase your intake too rapidly as it may cause flatulence and diarrhoea. Note that consuming very high levels of fibre may impede the absorption of certain vital minerals.

GI levels - quick clues

- **Sweetness:** is this food sweet? The sweeter it is, the more likely it is to have a high GI.
- **Fibre:** how much fibre is it likely to contain? The more, the better. If it's sweet but has no fibre, like a toffee or a sugar cube, then it definitely has a high GI. If it's sweet or sweetish but has some fibre (e.g., the peel on an apple, raspberries, dried apricots) then it's likely to have a low or medium GI. Fruit juice has an immediate impact on blood sugar.
- **Processing:** has it been processed? Processed food loses a lot of fibre (and other nutrients) in manufacturing and generally has a high GI.
- **Refining:** has it been refined? Refining foodstuffs such as flour also removes a lot of nutrients as well as fibre; white flour has the same very high GI as straight sugar. Go for wholegrains and wholegrain products, which are medium or low GI.

PROTEIN

Proteins are the building blocks of the human body. The cells of our bones, muscles, skin, nails, hair and every other tissue are made up of proteins, and proteins are needed to maintain them. They are also present in the blood and are needed to make new proteins (such as enzymes), and many other substances that allow the body to function. Proteins are made of amino acids, but not every source of protein contains all the amino acids that the body needs. The protein in our food is broken down into its component amino acids by the digestive system, and new proteins are synthesised by the body.

The best sources of protein in the diet are meat, fish, eggs, milk and other dairy products, tofu and soya products, quinoa, corn, lentils and other pulses. Protein obtained from animal sources is known as 'complete' protein because it contains all the amino acids that the body needs but cannot manufacture. Most protein that comes from plants is 'incomplete' and needs to be combined with other plant sources to get the full range, but soya and quinoa are complete proteins. Vegans in particular need to make sure they eat a good mix of pulses, nuts and seeds to get all the amino acids they need; vegetarians may get enough from dairy products and eggs.

Some people can eat too little and suffer from a protein deficiency. This can occur in vegans, but also in dieters – and it usually means that the latter have cut back on good sources of protein because of worries about fat levels. There is no need to do this, however: eggs, poultry, fish and low-fat dairy products can easily be incorporated into a weight-loss regime, and you do not have to exclude other sources completely as long as they are consumed in moderation and fit into your calorie allowance. Foods high in protein help you to feel full, too. Dairy products are particularly important because of the calcium they contain; do not be tempted to eliminate them. If the body does not get the calcium it needs from the diet, it will use calcium from its reserves – the bones. And some recent research also suggests calcium can have metabolic effects that actually encourage weight loss.

FAT

Fat was always considered the enemy when trying to lose weight. It's true that eating too much fat will lead to weight gain, but the emphasis in the last few decades on lowering fat levels and eating low-fat food has had no profound impact on weight levels overall. What is often obscured is the fact that fat is necessary.

Fat is a source of stored energy. It provides padding for the bones, it acts as insulation and keeps the body warm. It's needed in hormones, it forms part of every cell wall, and without fat some vitamins would be unavailable to the body because they're only fat soluble. On the other hand, fat – gram for gram – does contain more calories than protein or carbs. It is also not as easily used, meaning that it is more likely to be stored; hence the 'logic' of very low-fat diets. These have not proved to be sustainable (the extremely low-fat ones can even be dangerous), one reason being that fat gives food a lot of its flavour. To compensate for the lack of flavour, manufacturers of low-fat products have to add other ingredients, and that often means sugar. However, many of us still eat too much fat, and too much of the wrong sort. Not all fats are the same, and some are much better than others. It's important to cut the 'bad' fats and emphasise the 'good' ones. Cutting all fat is not necessary; being selective is.

Unsaturated fats are the ones to use; whether or not you are trying to lose weight, these will benefit your health. There are two basic types: monounsaturates and polyunsaturates. Olive and rapeseed oils are among the best sources of monounsaturates. There are two basic types of polyunsaturates: omega-3 and omega-6 essential fatty acids. These have to be obtained from food because the body cannot manufacture them, and while it's thought that most people get enough omega-6 in their diet at present, the same is not true for omega-3. The general recommendation is therefore to consume more foods containing high levels of omega-3. Good sources are cold-water oily fish such as salmon, herring, sardines and mackerel, as well as wheatgerm, linseeds, sesame seeds, and olive and rapeseed oils. It's also possible to buy eggs that have high levels of omega-3.

Saturated fats are the ones to cut back on. High levels of saturates have been shown to pose a risk to health, and it makes sense to moderate these. They are often of animal origin, with significant levels being found in meat and dairy products, although palm and coconut oils also contain high levels of saturates and are found in a wide range of processed foods. Trimming excess fat from meat and removing the skin from poultry are two basic measures that will cut both saturated fat and calories.

Trans fats (often called 'hydrogenated fats' or 'partly hydrogenated fats' on packaging) are the ones to try and eliminate; they are associated with significantly increased health risks, and are mainly found in processed food. These are liquid fats treated to make them solid at room temperature and are, consequently, much easier for the food industry to use. Many, but not all, manufacturers and fast-food chains are cutting down on their use of these fats.

Finally, note that for the vast majority of people cholesterol levels in the blood (cholesterol is a type of fat) are not affected by cholesterol levels in food. High levels of saturated fat make the difference, not the quantity of eggs eaten.

Fats in a nutshell

'Good' fats:

- Monounsaturates – olive and rapeseed oils; walnuts and avocados are also good sources. Use more.
- Omega-3 polyunsaturates – good sources include oily fish, linseeds, soya, and olive and rapeseed oils. Use more.
- Omega-6 polyunsaturates – sunflower and corn oils. No need to increase these deliberately.

'Bad' fats:

- Saturated fat – mostly of animal origin, includes lard, suet, meat, poultry skin, butter and other dairy products. Also in coconut and palm oils. Use less.
- Trans fats – also called hydrogenated or partly hydrogenated fats. Used in a lot of processed food. Avoid; check labels.

MICRONUTRIENTS

Vitamins, minerals and, recent evidence suggests, some phytochemicals – bioactive substances in plants – are needed by the body in small amounts to enable it to grow, develop and function. A diet containing plenty of fresh, unrefined foods should provide an adequate supply. Many of the processes used to manufacture and preserve foods can result in a loss of nutrients, and this is one of the reasons why large amounts of processed foods have no real place in a healthy diet.

Phytochemicals and antioxidants – many phytochemicals are antioxidants, though some, such as plant sterols, are not – have been getting a lot of attention lately. Antioxidants are powerful protective chemicals found in fruits and vegetables (some are manufactured in the body, too), which are needed in small amounts. Some are vitamins, such as vitamins A, C and E; others are minerals, such as selenium and zinc. Lycopene, found in tomatoes, is another; so is resveratrol, which is present in tea, grapes and red wine. Antioxidant supplements are available, but have not been shown to perform well; it's better to get them from food.

Here are the main vitamins and minerals, and the foods that are good sources of each.

Vitamin A

Liver, fish oils, eggs, butter, dark green, orange and yellow fruits and vegetables.
Essential for: strong bones, good vision, healthy skin, healing.

Vitamin B1 (Thiamine)

Animal and plant foods, especially wholegrain products; seafood, nuts, brown rice, soya beans.
Essential for: growth, nerve function, conversion of carbs and fats into energy.

Vitamin B2 (Riboflavin)

Liver, kidneys, milk and dairy products, green leafy vegetables, yeast.
Essential for: cell growth and reproduction, production of energy from carbohydrates.

Vitamin B3 (Niacin)

Meats, fish and poultry, wholegrains, peanuts, avocados.
Essential for: digestion, energy, the nervous system.

Vitamin B5 (Pantothenic acid)

Offal, fish, chicken, eggs, nuts, wholegrain cereals, mushrooms, pulses.

Essential for: strengthening immunity to disease and fighting infections, healing wounds.

Vitamin B6 (Pyridoxine)

Meat, eggs, wholegrains, yeast, cabbage, melon, molasses, potatoes, bananas.

Essential for: healthy immune system, production of antibodies, white blood cells and new cells.

Vitamin B12 (Cyanocolbalamin)

Beef, pork, lamb, offal, fish and seafood, dairy produce, eggs.

Essential for: energy and concentration, production of red blood cells, growth in children.

Note: vegetarians may need to take a supplement – long-term deficiency can cause irreversible nerve damage.

Folate

Liver, green vegetables, peas, beans and lentils, oranges.

Essential for: making DNA, normal growth and development, production of new cells.

Vitamin C

Fresh fruit and vegetables, potatoes, leafy herbs, berries.
Essential for: healthy skin, bones, muscles, healing, eyesight, protection from viruses.

Vitamin D

Oily fish, milk and dairy products, eggs.
Essential for: healthy teeth and bones, vital for growth.

Vitamin E

Eggs, milk, nuts, seeds, wholegrains, leafy vegetables, avocados, soya.
Essential for: absorption of iron and essential fatty acids, slowing the ageing process by protecting cells, increasing fertility.

Vitamin K

Cod liver oil, milk products, green vegetables, apricots, wholegrains.
Essential for: blood clotting.

Calcium

Fish where bones are eaten such as sardines, dairy produce, leafy green vegetables, nuts, root vegetables.
Essential for: strong bones and teeth, hormones and muscles, blood clotting, regulating blood pressure.

Iron

Red meat, liver, kidneys, shellfish, egg yolks, dark chocolate, cocoa powder, pulses, dark green vegetables, beans, dried fruit, molasses.
Essential for: transporting oxygen to the cells, health of the immune system.

Magnesium

Dark chocolate, brown rice, soya beans, nuts, wholegrains, pulses, legumes.
Essential for: transmission of nerve impulses, development of bones, growth and repair of cells, functioning of enzymes and metabolism in general.

Potassium

Dairy products, avocados, leafy green vegetables, bananas, fruit and vegetable juices, potatoes, nuts.

Essential for: maintaining water balance, nerve and muscle function.

DRINKS

Water is essential. Every part of the body needs it and it enables the body to absorb the vital nutrients from food. It also helps the digestive system to flush away waste products, and the general recommendation is to drink six to eight glasses a day. Soup is an excellent way of combining food and water, and can keep you feeling full for a long time – a great tip when you're dieting.

Water is at least calorie-free; the same cannot be said of many other drinks, and there is a tendency to forget about them when counting calories. There are other factors that should also be considered. Sugary carbonated drinks are coming under suspicion because of the high-fructose corn syrup they often contain. As with fats, it's beginning to become clear that not all sugars behave in the same way, at least as far as their effects on health are concerned.

The major problem with tea and coffee, where weight loss is concerned, is the milk and sugar that are often added (though caffeine also has an effect on insulin levels). If you take milk with your hot drinks, reduce the amount and change to skimmed milk – good advice generally – or try black coffee and herbal teas. Try weaning yourself off sugar if you can; in the long term it is better to try and change the habit rather than accommodate it with sweeteners.

Remember that alcohol dehydrates you as well as bumping up your calorie total without providing any nutritional value. If you drink two small (175ml – glass sizes have increased, so watch this) glasses of red wine a day, you're consuming nearly 250 empty calories. A pint of beer can be around 180 to 200. Drink extra water during and after drinking alcohol to avoid the effects of dehydration (one of the causes of hangovers).

A BALANCED DIET?
Knowing theoretically what is good and what is not, and putting at least some of it into practice, is one thing. Assessing the overall balance of your diet can be more difficult, and it is here that errors and assumptions can easily be made.

In the US, the government has developed the 'Food Pyramid' to help with this balance. Versions of this 'pyramid' are available from many other sources, but they can be difficult to understand and implement, and many scientists have been critical of the balance of foods they suggest. There are also several types of plate diagrams – which use a plate divided into sections by food type – but again these are awkward to apply to your diet as a whole. This diversity of recommendation has led to the idea that scientists change their minds a great deal, but this is not actually the case. The basic advice remains essentially the same:

Concentrate on eating a wide variety of vegetables and fruits.

Eat bread, rice, pasta and other starchy foods but – and note the but – choose wholegrain types as much as possible. This means, for example, eating brown rice and wholemeal bread rather than white rice and white bread. Potatoes are acceptable, though filling up on them is not advised.

Consume milk and other dairy products (less than half the above categories in quantity).

Consume some non-dairy sources of protein: meat, fish, eggs, beans, etc. (in about the same quantities as dairy products).
Only consume a very little – or none at all – of the foods and drinks that are high in sugar and fat.

A balanced meal would consist of more vegetables and wholegrains than meat, for example, and a cheese sandwich would be a more balanced lunch if it included some salad, was accompanied with a couple of tomatoes and was followed by an apple. You could then use less cheese, too.

The aim, however, is to achieve an overall balance. If you keep a food diary you will get a general idea; you would be able to spot a creeping tendency to eat too much bread, eat meat at every meal or drink a lot of milk. A few tweaks, and the balance is back. It's important not to get bogged down in trying to achieve perfection (which would be impossible) or be so despondent that you abandon the whole idea. When you are calorie counting it's important to make every calorie count, so try and get it roughly right.

Healthy eating shortcuts

- Eat as many differently coloured fruits and vegetables as you can each day, increasing the range of vitamins you get.
- Keep foods such as bread, pasta and rice low or medium GI, using wholegrain and unrefined alternatives wherever possible.
- Fill up with fibre and drink plenty of water to bulk it up – this will help the digestive system work efficiently and keep you feeling full for longer.
- Opt for lean protein sources, and keep saturated fats to a minimum.

Salt

Excess salt in the diet raises blood pressure and increases the risk of heart disease and strokes. In the UK, we consume around 9g per person a day; most of this comes from processed foods rather than from salt added during home cooking or at the table. Experts recommend reducing salt intake to 1.5g a day.

COOKING METHODS

Cooking is one way of immediately making the food you eat more nutritious and more diet-friendly, and existing recipes can usually be adapted. Preparing your own food is nothing but good news when trying to lose weight, not just because you control the ingredients, but also because you determine the cooking method. The way you cook food will affect both its calorie content and its nutritional value, so it makes sense to employ the best methods and use some tricks of the trade:

Any fats added during cooking, such as oil for frying or a knob of butter on top, will add to the calorie count of the final dish. Young boiled carrots contain 22 calories per 100g. A small knob of butter – say 5g – on top would add another 37 calories. Measure oils and fats, as errors and false assumptions can make a big difference. Using spoon measures will really help.

Sugar added during cooking will also increase calorie content: 100g of apples stewed without sugar contain just 35 calories, while 100g stewed with some sugar contain more than double that amount, at 74 calories. Again, measuring is vital.

Non-stick pans dramatically reduce the need for oil when frying. Where two tablespoons might be necessary in an ordinary pan, cooking in a non-stick pan could reduce that amount to two teaspoons – a difference of 180 calories. When you boil vegetables, vitamins and minerals leach out into the cooking water; steaming, stir-frying or cooking briefly in a microwave retains more of these vital nutrients. Stir-frying also requires a minimal amount of oil if you use a non-stick wok.

Soups, stews and casseroles preserve more of the nutritional value of foods, as vitamins and minerals are retained in the liquid. There is also evidence that soups, in particular, help you to feel full for longer, thus reducing the tendency to snack.

Keep fibre content as high as possible. This means doing things such as leaving the skin on potatoes or apples, and using wholemeal flour or pasta whenever you can.

Grilling meat on a rack that allows fat to drip through will reduce the fat content. A fried rump steak has 190 calories per 100g, while grilled rump steak has only 168 caiories per 100g.

Dry-frying is another useful cooking method, especially for bacon. Do not add any fat to the pan, but simply fry the bacon in its own fat and drain it well once cooked. Draining it on kitchen roll reduces the fat level further.

In general, the shorter the cooking time, the more nutrients will be retained, and the fewer fats or sugars added, the lower the calorie count.

PORTION SIZES

Over time, portion sizes have increased almost without us noticing; we have become used to being served more and more, and research has shown that people given big portions will tend to eat more than they actually need. Calorie counting really helps with portion control, but when you start you may feel that the quantity of something you weigh and allow for – 100g of pasta, for example – is much less than you think you might want. If you find this happening, there are several things you can do:

Use a smaller plate. Surprisingly, perhaps, plate sizes have also increased and a normal helping does not look right on an outsized plate. Using a smaller plate will make your helping seem more filling – and this is supported by scientific evidence. (Glass sizes have also increased, and even smaller wine glasses now hold 175ml, so be careful there, too.)

Have a salad with every meal. Providing that lots of high-calorie, high-fat dressings are not included, this is a great way of adding nutrients and fibre to a meal and making it more satisfying.

Check the balance of your meal and add more vegetables, cooked in the most low-calorie way.

Try wholemeal alternatives in the case of, for instance, pasta. They will be more satisfying.

Pasta, rice and pulses

Note that pasta, rice and pulses swell to up to approximately three times their weight when cooked. Food packaging may often give values for dry weight. Note that 100g of boiled white rice has 138 calories, but 100g of dry uncooked rice has 343 calories; 100g of standard cooked pasta has 89 calories, while 100g of the same uncooked pasta has 362 calories. In practice, 100g of pasta or rice is a good portion; 80g may be enough.

Calorie shortcuts

With a little time, and repeated weighing, you will quickly get to know some calorie values off by heart. Here are a few rough shortcuts in the meantime (all spoon measures are level; heaped spoonfuls can contain twice as much). Continue, however, to weigh or measure high-calorie items.

Almonds – about 13 calories a nut.

Apples – a medium apple is between 50–55 calories. A medium cooking apple is 70 calories.

Apricots – fresh, 16 calories; dried, average, 10.

Asparagus – six or seven spears are 25 calories.

Avocado – half a medium avocado is approximately 160 calories.

Bacon – two thick rashers of back bacon are about 100g raw weight. Dry-fried, their weight drops to 35g, 103 calories.

Beer – on average, a pint is 184 calories and lagers are about 166.

Brazil nuts – 25 calories per nut.

Bread – slices vary in thickness and size, so weigh at first and make a mental note. The same applies to rolls.

Breakfast cereals – a standard helping is 30–35g. As with bread, weigh it first.

Butter – weigh carefully, but allow 40 calories for a teaspoon.

Cashew nuts – about 15 calories per complete nut.

Cheese – high in calories, so weigh.

Chutneys and pickles – per tablespoon, mango chutney is about 60 calories, sweet pickle is 28, an average fruit chutney is 38 and piccalilli is 17.

Cider – a half pint of dry cider is 99 calories; with sweet cider that rises to 116 and vintage can be as high as 270.

Dates – per dried date, 27 calories.

Eggs – small hen's egg, 70 calories; medium, 80–85; large, 100.

Grapefruit – half, 30 calories.

Hazelnuts – 8 nuts are about 10g and 65 calories.

Honey – 25 calories for a level (as far as possible) teaspoon.

Jam – allow 20–25 calories for a teaspoon.

Kiwi fruit – average, 39 calories.

Mayonnaise – per tablespoon: extra light, 15; light or reduced-calorie, 45; standard, 105.

Milk – a tablespoon is roughly the quantity most people use in tea or coffee, and is 10 calories for full-cream milk, 5 for skimmed.

Nectarine – average fruit, 48–50 calories.

Oil – allow 40–45 per teaspoon and 120–135 per tablespoon.

Olives – allow 5 calories per stuffed olive and 3 for unstuffed ones.

Onions – a medium onion, topped and tailed, is about 100g and 36 calories.

Peaches – average fruit, 40 calories.

Peanut butter – a teaspoon of smooth peanut butter has 30 calories.

Peanuts – weigh, as they can be an addictive snack (avoid salted ones)!

Pears – average fruit, 64 calories.

Peppers – an average sweet pepper, deseeded, weighs 100g, so 15 calories for green; 28 for yellow and 32 for orange or red.

Pickled onions – one, on average, is 10 calories.

Pistachios – 30 calories for 10 shelled nuts.

Plums – a large one is 36 calories.

Potatoes – weigh; rough sizes can be deceptive.

Raspberries – 100g is a large helping and 25 calories.

Rice, cooked – as a guide, allow 30 calories per level tablespoon of boiled white rice. Where possible, weigh.

Spirits – all have 56 calories to a 25ml standard bar measure, but it's easy to pour double that.

Spring onions – five trimmed spring onions are 6 calories.

Strawberries – an average helping is about 100g and 27 calories.

Sugar – 20 calories per teaspoon (or cube).

Syrups – golden syrup, 45 calories per tablespoon; maple syrup, 52.

Tomato ketchup – 18 calories per tablespoon.

Tomato purée – 12 calories per tablespoon.

Tomatoes – large, about 17 calories.

Walnuts – 50 calories for a whole large walnut.

Wine – per 175ml glass: red, 119; rosé, 124; dry white, 116; medium and sparkling white, 130.

How to use the *Calorie Counter*

The foods in this book are grouped into categories – Bakery, Biscuits, Dairy, etc. – and listed in bold type in alphabetical order in the left-hand column of each page together with the name of the manufacturer of branded foods. The energy value in calories, the protein, carbohydrate and fat contents per 100g or 100ml are given in the second and third, fourth, fifth and sixth columns respectively. This enables you to compare across types of food and brands, etc., but to find the values for a 28g portion of cheese, you would have to divide the figures given by 100 and multiply by 28. Where we have been unable to obtain the information per 100g/100ml, this has been specified. Here it should be noted that manufacturers often amend portion sizes; if in doubt, check on the packaging.

Values for unbranded foods have been obtained from *The Composition of Foods* (5th edition, 1991; and 6th summary edition, 2002) and *Vegetables, Herbs and Spices* (supplement, 1991), and have been reproduced by permission of Controller of Her Majesty's Stationery Office. Where we had gaps, we consulted the websites of the major retailers, as well as www.mysupermarket.co.uk. We also wish to thank the staff in various branches of Morrisons, Holland & Barrett and the Co-Operative for their assistance.

Key to reading the tables

The publishers are grateful to all the manufacturers who gave information on their products. The list of foods included is as up-to-date as it was possible to make it, but it should be remembered that new products are frequently put on the market and existing ones withdrawn or recipes amended, so it has not been possible to include everything. If you cannot find a particular food here, you can still, however, obtain guideline figures by finding an equivalent product from one of the other manufacturers listed in the book.

g:	gram
Cal:	calorie (the same as kCal)
kCal:	kilocalorie
ml:	millilitre
N:	the nutrient is present in significant quantities but there is no accurate information on the precise amount available
n/a:	not available
Tr:	trace (less than 0.1g present)
as sold:	usually refers to mixes, granules, etc., which need to have milk or water added

Food Type

	cal per 100g	cal per portion	pro (g)	carb (g)	fat (g)

Bakery

Non-Branded Bread and Rolls

Bread

	cal per 100g	cal per portion	pro (g)	carb (g)	fat (g)
brown	207		7.9	42.1	2
brown, toasted	272		10.4	56.5	2.1
ciabatta	271		10.2	52	3.9
currant	289		7.5	50.7	7.6
currant, toasted	323		8.4	56.8	8.5
Danish style	228		9.1	44.5	2.7
French stick	263		9	56.1	1.9
garlic bread, pre-packed, frozen	365		7.8	45	18.3
granary	237		9.6	47.4	2.3
malt, fruited	295		7.8	64.9	2.3
muffins, white	262		10.4	41.6	6
muffins, wholemeal	219		10.8	36.2	3.4
pitta, white	255		9.1	55.1	1.3
rye	219		8.3	45.8	1.7
wheatgerm	220		11.1	39.5	3.1
wheatgerm, toasted	271		12.1	53.2	2.6
white (sliced)	219		7.9	46.1	1.6
white, fried in oil/lard	498		8.1	46.8	32.2
white, toasted	267		9.7	56.2	2
wholemeal	217		9.4	42	2.5
wholemeal, toasted	255		11.2	49.2	2.9

Food Type	cal per 100g	cal per portion	pro (g)	carb (g)	fat (g)
Rolls					
brown, crusty	255		10.3	50.4	2.8
brown, soft	236		9.9	44.8	3.2
granary	238		10.2	42.7	4.2
hamburger buns	264		9.1	48.8	5
white, crusty	262		9.2	54.9	2.2
white, soft	254		9.3	51.5	2.6
wholemeal	244		10.4	46.1	3.3
Branded Bread and Rolls					
Bagels NEW YORK BAGEL CO.					
cinnamon & raisin	253		7.7	51.1	2
fruit 'n oats	264		8.9	52.3	2.1
multi-seeded	263		13.9	37.1	6.5
onion	261		9.3	49	3.1
plain	255		9.1	50.4	1.9
seeded bran	269		11.6	37.4	8.1
sesame	266		10.3	49.2	3.1
Bread					
50/50 KINGSMILL	225		9.9	41.2	2.3
50/50 with Omega 3 KINGSMILL	225		9.9	41.2	2.3
All in One WARBURTON	225		10.3	41	1.8
Best of Both HOVIS	214		9	40.4	1.8
Best of Both Invisible Crust HOVIS	214		9	40.4	1.8

Food Type	cal per 100g	cal per portion	pro (g)	carb (g)	fat (g)
Buckwheat, organic ARTISAN BREAD ORIGINAL	184		6.1	38.1	1.8
Crusts Away! 50/50 KINGSMILL	204		8.8	37.7	2
Crusts Away! White KINGSMILL	222		8	43.3	1.9
Crusty White WARBURTON	249		10.6	46.5	2.3
Danish Brown WEIGHTWATCHERS	215		11	38.8	1.8
Danish Malted WEIGHTWATCHERS	241		12.4	44.5	1.6
Danish White WARBURTON	243		10.7	46.9	1.3
Danish White WEIGHTWATCHERS	238		10.5	45.8	1.2
Essene, organic ARTISAN BREAD ORIGINAL	199		7.7	38.1	1.8
Farmhouse Best of Both HOVIS	225		9.5	42.1	2
Farmhouse White HOVIS	234		8.7	44.6	2.3
Farmhouse Wholemeal HOVIS	216		10	37.8	2.7
Gold Farmhouse White KINGSMILL	236		8.4	44.7	2.6
Gold Seeds & Oats Soft & Crunchy KINGSMILL	287		11.1	40.1	9.1
Gold Seeds & Oats Wholesome & Nutty KINGSMILL	282		11.3	41.2	8
Granary Original HOVIS	248		10.3	46.4	2.4
Granary White HOVIS	233		9.7	40.8	3.5
Granary Wholemeal HOVIS	223		10.6	39.8	2.4
Great Everyday White KINGSMILL	232		9	44.6	2
Healthy Inside WARBURTON	230		10.8	41.2	2.4

Food Type	cal per 100g	cal per portion	pro (g)	carb (g)	fat (g)
Linseed, organic ARTISAN BREAD					
ORIGINAL	222		6.4	42	4.3
Little Brown Loaf HOVIS	216		10	37.8	2.7
Malted Harvestgrain Batch					
ALLINSON	244		9.9	45.2	2.6
Malted Wholegrain NIMBLE	222		10.4	41.9	1.4
Muffins, white KINGSMILL	224		9.8	42.3	1.7
Original Wheatgerm HOVIS	214		10	38.6	2.2
Premium Brown WARBURTON	249		10.6	43.2	3.7
Pumpernickel, organic BIONA	182		6.8	36	1.2
Rice, organic ARTISAN BREAD ORIGINAL	216		4.9	44.9	1.9
Rye Amaranth/Quinoa BIONA	176		4.9	34.2	2.2
Rye with Sunflower Seeds,					
organic SUNNYVALE	198		5.1	30.3	6.3
San Francisco Sour Dough					
LOYD GROSSMAN	249		9	50.5	1.2
Scottish Plain Batch SUNBLEST	233		10.1	42.3	2.6
Seed Sensations Light &					
Nutty HOVIS	258		10.1	43.6	4.8
Seed Sensations Rich &					
Roasted HOVIS	255		10	42	5.3
Seeded Batch WARBURTON	288		12.3	39.7	8.9
Soya & Linseed Bread BURGEN	274		15.9	29.8	10.1
Spelt, organic AMISA	291		7	36	n/a
Spelt, Focaccia, organic AMISA	291		8.2	54.1	4.4

Food Type	cal per 100g	cal per portion	pro (g)	carb (g)	fat (g)
Stoneground Wholemeal					
WARBURTON	210		10.3	35.7	2.6
Sunflower & Pumpkin Batch					
ALLINSON	279		11.8	38.7	8.5
Tasty Wholemeal KINGSMILL	227		10.5	37.7	3.8
Toastie KINGSMILL	232		9	44.6	2
Toastie, White (400g) WARBURTON	275		10.3	45.1	1.9
Toastie, White (800g) WARBURTON	234		9.9	43.8	2
White Farmhouse (400g)					
WARBURTON	239		10.1	43.7	2.6
White Farmhouse (800g)					
WARBURTON	236		9.9	43.4	2.5
White NIMBLE	219		10.1	40.6	1.8
White SUNBLEST	228		8	45.7	1.5
White, medium slice (400g)					
WARBURTON	239		10.3	45.1	1.9
White, medium slice (800g)					
WARBURTON	234		9.9	43.8	2
White, soft HOVIS	234		8.7	44.6	2.3
White, thick slice (400g)					
WARBURTON	237		10.4	48.6	0.8
Wholegrain & Cranberry BURGEN	234		10.7	37.1	4.7
Wholegrain Goodness WARBURTON	232		10.9	38.4	3.9
Wholemeal Batch ALLINSON	219		10.5	37	3.2
Wholemeal HOVIS	216		10	37.8	2.7

Food Type	cal per 100g	cal per portion	pro (g)	carb (g)	fat (g)
Wholemeal NIMBLE	219		12.2	37	2.5
Wholemeal (400g) WARBURTON	231		10.4	40.7	2.5
Wholemeal (800g) WARBURTON	231		10.2	39.6	2.5
Wholemeal, fibre boost					
WARBURTON	202		10.1	34.7	2.6
Wholemeal, organic HOVIS	211		8.8	37.9	2.7
Chapatis					
made with fat	328		8.1	48.3	12.8
made without fat	202		7.3	43.7	1
plain PATAK	280		8	48.1	6.1
plain, mini LOYD GROSSMAN	255		11	45	3.5
Milk Roll					
white WARBURTON	249		11	45	2.8
Naan Bread	285		7.8	50.2	7.3
Garlic & Coriander PATAK	277		8.9	46.2	6.3
Garlic & Coriander SHARWOOD	272		8.5	42.9	7.4
Peshwari SHARWOOD	257		7.2	45.1	5.3
Plain PATAK	277		8.9	46.7	6
Plain SHARWOOD	272		8.1	48	5.1
Pitta Bread					
plain	250		10	50	1
Plain, white LOYD GROSSMAN	265		9.7	48.7	3.5
Plain, wholemeal LOYD GROSSMAN	252		9.9	45.1	3.5
Rice Flour Pancakes					
BLUE DRAGON	340		5.8	77.4	0.5

Food Type	cal per 100g	cal per portion	pro (g)	carb (g)	fat (g)
Rolls					
50/50 KINGSMILL	236		9.3	41.2	3.8
Best of Both HOVIS	238		10.7	37.4	5
Malted WEIGHTWATCHERS	251		11.7	47.1	1.8
Malted Grain WARBURTON	269		10.9	43.3	4.3
malted white	251		11.7	47.1	1.8
Seeded WARBURTON	314		13.3	41.2	8.7
Tasty Wholemeal KINGSMILL	232		10.6	38.8	3.8
White KINGSMILL	248		8.9	46.7	2.8
White, Lunch WARBURTON	249		10.8	40.8	3.2
White, Sliced WARBURTON	258		9.7	44.6	4.5
White, Soft WARBURTON	264		11	45	4.4
Wholemeal, Lunch WARBURTON	233		10.7	2.8	3.2
Wholemeal, Sliced WARBURTON	220		10.5	35.8	3.9
Wholemeal, Soft WARBURTON	227		10.9	35	4.7
Spring Roll Wrappers					
BLUE DRAGON	340		5.8	77.4	0.5
Taco Shells					
DISCOVERY FOODS	489		5.7	53.4	28.1
OLD EL PASO	506		7	61	26
Tortillas					
Corn OLD EL PASO	343		10	60	7
Flour OLD EL PASO	344		8.7	51.1	11.7
Flour, Salsa Flavour OLD EL PASO	323		9	52	9

Food Type	cal per 100g	cal per portion	pro (g)	carb (g)	fat (g)
Garlic & Coriander, Wheat					
DISCOVERY FOODS	289		8.1	50.8	6
Plain, Wheat DISCOVERY FOODS	478		6.6	68.1	24
Wholemeal, Wheat DISCOVERY					
FOODS	273		9.2	40.4	8.3
Wraps					
Multi-Seed DISCOVERY FOODS	303		89	54.2	5.6
White DISCOVERY FOODS	279		9.1	49.6	4.9
Wholemeal DISCOVERY FOODS	273		9.2	40.4	8.3
Breakfast & Teatime					
Breads/Cakes					
Blueberry Muffin	327		7	50	11
Chocolate Muffin					
Galaxy MCVITIES	446		5.2	50.3	24.9
mini FLETCHERS	420		5.3	47.3	22.8
Croissants	425		9	41	25
Crumpets					
KINGSMILL	180		5.8	37.5	0.8
MOTHER'S PRIDE	187		5.6	38.9	1
WARBURTON	173		5.6	36.1	0.7
Croissants					
mini DELIFRANCE	316		6.5	37.4	16
Currant Buns	280		8	52.6	5.6
Danish Pastries	342		5.8	51.3	14.1

Food Type	cal per 100g	cal per portion	pro (g)	carb (g)	fat (g)
Doughnuts					
jam	336		5.7	48.8	14.5
ring	403		6.1	47.2	22.4
Eccles Cakes	387		4	56.3	17.8
LANCASHIRE ECCLES CAKES LTD	424		4.2	64.1	16.8
Fruit Loaf					
cinnamon & raisin SOREEN	307		7	63.8	2.2
Lincolnshire plum SOREEN	261		8.4	49.3	3.4
with orange WARBURTON	245		7.4	48.2	2.5
Fruity Teacakes					
WARBURTON	256		8.7	48	3.3
Hot Cross Buns	312		7.4	58.4	7
white KINGSMILL	261		9.1	48.2	3.5
Lemon Muffin					
mini FLETCHERS	370		4.3	50.7	16.3
Malt Loaf					
Fruity, Original SOREEN	310		7.4	65.6	2
Pain au Chocolat	420		8	43	24
Pancakes					
AUNT BESSIE'S	150		6.1	24.6	3.1
KINGSMILL	264		5.5	51	4.2
WARBURTON	239		7.6	37.7	6.4
Potato Cakes					
WARBURTON	260		4.7	37.5	10.1

Food Type	cal per 100g	cal per portion	pro (g)	carb (g)	fat (g)
Raisin Loaf with Cinnamon					
WARBURTON	267		7.2	51.1	3.7
Scones					
sultana	344		8	51	12
wholemeal	328		8.8	43	14.6
Scotch Pancakes	270		5.6	43	9.6
Soda Farls					
IRWIN'S RANKIN	223		4	44	3.4
Waffles					
MCVITIE'S	470		5.9	53.9	25.7
Belgian Chocolate, organic					
DOVES FARM	456		7.3	55.2	22.9
Waffles, Spelt					
organic DOVES FARM	429		7.8	49.1	22.4
Cakes & Cream Cakes					
Almond Cake Slice					
WEIGHTWATCHERS	365		5.2	63.8	9.9
Almond Slices					
MR KIPLING	415		6.4	64.1	14.8
Apple Crumble Slice					
WEIGHTWATCHERS	346		0.5	64.8	7.7
Angel Slices					
MR KIPLING	418		2.7	60.1	18.5
Apple Slices, Delightful					
MR KIPLING	300		4.4	63.4	3.2

Food Type	cal per 100g	cal per portion	pro (g)	carb (g)	fat (g)
Bakewell Slices					
MR KIPLING	447		4.3	64.4	19.2
Battenburg Cake					
LYONS CAKES	433		6.3	73.7	11.4
MR KIPLING	427		6.1	72.7	12.4
mini LYONS CAKES	450		4.9	81.2	11.8
Caramel Cake Bars					
CADBURY	370		4	47.5	18
WEIGHTWATCHERS	377		5.6	58.2	13.5
Caramel Shortcake					
WEIGHTWATCHERS	484		5.2	57.6	25.9
Carrot Cake					
FRÜ	354		3.8	45.3	17.5
organic RESPECT	400		3	47.8	22.6
Carrot Cake Slices					
WEIGHTWATCHERS	263		3	56.7	2.7
Carrot & Walnut Mini Classic					
MR KIPLING	439		4.5	48.6	25.2
Chocolate Bites					
GÜ	480		3.8	51.9	28.3
Chocolate Cake Bars					
CADBURY	430		5.4	54	21.6
LYONS CAKES	433		4.7	54.3	21.9
MCVITIE'S	360		5.5	54.9	13.2

Food Type	cal per 100g	cal per portion	pro (g)	carb (g)	fat (g)
THORNTON'S	437		5	50.5	24
WEIGHTWATCHERS	372		5.6	53.5	15.1
Chocolate Chip Cake Bars					
MCVITIE'S	360		5.5	54.9	13.2
MR KIPLING	470		5.3	53.5	26.3
Chocolate Cup Cakes					
FABULOUS BAKIN' BOYS	448		4	54	24
LYONS CAKES	375		2.5	71.4	8.8
mini WEIGHTWATCHERS	422		6.1	52	21.1
Chocolate Slices					
MR KIPLING	405		5.5	51.3	19.8
Chocolate Slices, Belgian					
WEIGHTWATCHERS	329		5.9	61.3	6.7
Chocolate Slices, Delightful					
MR KIPLING	307		6.2	56.2	6.4
Coconut Sponge Sandwich Cake	400		3.6	56.9	17.3
Country Slices					
MR KIPLING	384		4.4	56.9	15.4
Country Slices, Delightful					
MR KIPLING	315		4.1	63.6	4.9
Date & Walnut Cake Slices					
WEIGHTWATCHERS	271		3.5	60.6	1.6
Eclairs					
frozen	396		5.6	26.1	30.6
WEIGHTWATCHERS	271		3.9	37.4	11.7

Food Type	cal per 100g	cal per portion	pro (g)	carb (g)	fat (g)
Fancy Iced Cakes	355		3.8	68.8	9.1
Flake Cake CADBURY	445		5.4	46.5	26.6
Flapjack					
standard	493		4.8	62.4	27
Apple & Sultana, organic					
DOVES FARM	446		4.7	61.1	19.6
Bakewell JULIAN GRAVES	438		6.1	58.2	20
Butter, organic DOVES FARM	432		6.1	59.4	18.8
Chocolate FABULOUS BAKIN' BOYS	494		6.3	61.8	24.6
Chocolate JULIAN GRAVES	434		6.9	56.7	19.9
Fruit JULIAN GRAVES	405		6.9	58.6	15.9
Goji Berry JULIAN GRAVES	407		6.8	59.4	15.7
Golden Oaty FABULOUS BAKIN' BOYS	465		5.6	59	23
Hobnob MCVITIE'S	449		5.7	59.4	21
Hobnob Chocolate MCVITIE'S	454		5.7	59.5	21.4
Original JULIAN GRAVES	414		7.2	57.9	16.9
Toffee JULIAN GRAVES	432		6.7	58.5	19
Yoghurt JULIAN GRAVES	438		6.6	58.1	19.8
French Fancies					
MR KIPLING	378		2.6	69.7	2.7
Fruit Cake					
plain, retail	371		5.1	57.9	14.8
rich, iced	350		3.6	65.9	9.8
wholemeal	366		6	52.4	16.2
MCVITIE'S	367		4.6	55.3	14.2

Food Type	cal per 100g	cal per portion	pro (g)	carb (g)	fat (g)
Fudge Cake Bars					
CADBURY	420		5.7	60.3	17.6
Galaxy Cake Bars					
MCVITIE'S	491		4.7	55.3	27.9
Gâteau, Double Chocolate	302		4.7	28	19
Genoa Cake	299		3.8	53	8
Golden Syrup Cake Bars					
MCVITIE'S	355		3.4	60.4	11
Jaffa Cake Bars					
MCVITIE'S	408		4	58.5	17.5
Jamaica Ginger Cake Bars					
MCVITIE'S	393		3.4	61.9	16.6
Lemon Cake Bars					
MCVITIE'S	392		4.5	54.8	17.2
Lemon Cake Slices					
WEIGHTWATCHERS	304		3.7	68.8	1.6
Lemon Slices					
MR KIPLING	413		4.1	61.9	16.6
Madeira Cake	388		5	56	16
cherry	286		4.4	42	11
Manor House Cake					
MR KIPLING	400		5.2	50.5	19.7
Milky Way Cake Bars					
MCVITIE'S	511		5	53.8	30.6
Millionaire's Shortbread	507		2.9	61.9	27.5

Food Type	cal per 100g	cal per portion	pro (g)	carb (g)	fat (g)
Mini Rolls					
Caramel CADBURY	435		5.1	57.1	20.8
Chocolate CADBURY	445		4.9	56	22.5
Chocolate MARS	433		5.1	61.4	18.5
Chocolate WEIGHTWATCHERS	334		4.6	58.1	13.2
Jaffa Cakes MCVITIE'S	382		3.5	67.2	11
Jam CADBURY	420		2.4	59.6	18.5
Mint Crisp Cake Bars					
CADBURY	440		4.1	55.1	22.9
Orange Crisp Cake Bars					
CADBURY	440		4.1	54.8	23
Pecan Cup Cakes	420		3.3	52.1	22.3
Sponge Cake					
dairy cream-filled	295		3.7	43	12
fatless	301		10	53	6.9
jam-filled	302		4.2	64.2	4.9
Swiss Gâteau					
CADBURY	425		4.9	59.6	18.7
Swiss Roll					
chocolate, individual	386		4.3	58.1	16.8
Chocolate, jumbo LYONS CAKES	403		3.8	54.5	18.9
Raspberry MR KIPLING	335		3	65	6.9
Raspberry & Vanilla, jumbo LYONS CAKES	366		2.9	60.8	12.4
Trifle Sponges	338		4.5	73.5	2.9

Food Type	cal per 100g	cal per portion	pro (g)	carb (g)	fat (g)
Triple Choc' Roll					
CADBURY	360		4.6	51.6	15.1
Vanilla Cake Bars					
CADBURY	475		3.7	54.5	26.8
Victoria Mini Classics					
MR KIPLING	419		3.8	58.7	18.8
Victoria Slices					
MR KIPLING	445		4.6	70	16.3
Victoria Sponges					
mini WEIGHTWATCHERS	354		5.7	64.1	8.3
Pies, Tarts & Pastries					
Apple Strudel					
COPPENWRATH & WEISE	241		3	25.8	14
Bakewell Tart					
LYONS CAKES	388		3.9	54.6	17.1
Bramley Apple Pie					
AUNT BESSIE'S	255		2.8	36.2	11
MR KIPLING	344		3.3	54.1	12.7
Bramley Apple & Blackberry Pie					
AUNT BESSIE'S	256		2.6	38	10.3
Bramley Apple & Blackcurrant Pies					
MR KIPLING	345		3.3	54.2	12.7
Cherry Bakewells	404		3.8	59	17
gluten-free	374		1.4	61.1	13.8

Food Type	cal per 100g	cal per portion	pro (g)	carb (g)	fat (g)
MR KIPLING	426		3.9	61.4	18.4
Custard Tarts	269		9	29	13
Dutch Apple Turnovers	395		3.5	59.4	16.7
Fruit Pie					
individual	356		4.3	56.7	14
one crust	190		2.1	28.8	8.2
wholemeal, one crust	185		2.7	26.5	8.3
Fruit Strudel					
COPPENWRATH & WEISE	273		3.8	30.3	15.2
Fruity Pies					
selection MR KIPLING	346		3.3	54.6	12.7
Jam Tarts					
assorted	402		2.8	64	15
MR KIPLING	383		3.5	63.6	12.8
Lemon Curd Tarts	402		2.8	64	15
Lemon Meringue Pie					
standard	251		2.9	43.5	8.5
AUNT BESSIE'S	271		3.4	58.8	2.5
Morello Cherry Pie					
AUNT BESSIE'S	274		2.8	41.7	10.6
Summer Fruits Lattice Tart					
AUNT BESSIE'S					
Treacle Lattice Tart					
LYONS CAKES	379		4.2	63.4	12.1
Treacle Tart	379		3.9	62.8	14.2

Food Type	cal per 100g	cal per portion	pro (g)	carb (g)	fat (g)
Beans, Lentils & Cereals					
Beans & Lentils					
Aduki Beans					
dried	272		19.9	50.1	0.5
dried, boiled	123		9.3	22.5	0.2
canned, organic BIONA	130		7.5	24.8	0.1
canned, organic EPICURE	128		19.9	7.5	0.1
Black Beans					
canned, organic BIONA	132		8.8	23.7	0.4
canned, organic EPICURE	91		6.1	16.6	0.3
Blackeye Beans					
dried	311		23.5	54.1	1.6
dried, boiled	116		8.8	19.9	0.7
canned, organic BIONA	455		7	18.5	0.1
Broad Beans					
canned	82		8	11	
Butter Beans					
canned	77		5.9	13	0.5
dried, boiled	103		7.1	18.4	0.6
canned, organic BIONA	101		16.8	n/a	0.6
canned, organic EPICURE	80		5.9	13	0.5
Cannellini Beans					
canned	87		7	14	0.3
canned, organic EPICURE	84		6.8	17.9	2.8

Food Type	cal per 100g	cal per portion	pro (g)	carb (g)	fat (g)
Chickpeas					
canned	115		7.2	16.1	2.9
dried	320		21.3	49.6	5.4
dried, boiled	121		8.4	18.2	2.1
canned, organic BIONA	118		8.4	16.6	2.1
canned, organic EPICURE	119		7.2	16.1	0.4
Chilli Beans					
canned	80		4.8	14	0.5
dried	70		4.9	12.2	0.5
Haricot Beans					
canned	69		7	9	0.5
dried	286		21.4	49.7	1.6
dried, boiled	95		6.6	17.2	0.5
canned, organic BIONA	94		6.6	15.7	0.5
canned, organic EPICURE	95		6.6	7.2	0.5
Lentils					
green/brown, dried	297		24.3	48.8	1.9
green/brown, dried, boiled	105		8.8	16.9	0.7
green, canned, organic BIONA	103		8.8	15.4	0.7
Puy style, as sold JULIAN GRAVES	342		28.1	57.1	0.1
Puy style, canned MERCHANT GOURMET	118		7.7	0.3	21.1
Puy style, dried MERCHANT GOURMET	307		24.6	49.4	1.2
red, split, dried	318		23.8	56.3	1.3

Food Type	cal per 100g	cal per portion	pro (g)	carb (g)	fat (g)
red, split, dried, boiled	100		7.6	17.5	0.4
red, split, as sold, JULIAN GRAVES	342		28.1	57.1	0.1
Marrowfat Peas					
canned	84		6	14	0.4
Bigga, canned BATCHELORS	75		5.6	11.8	0.6
Farrow's Giant, canned					
BATCHELORS	77		5.9	12.3	0.5
Marrowfat Peas, Dried					
Bigga, as sold BATCHELORS	84		8.3	10.3	1.1
as sold WHITWORTHS	298		21.6	50	1.3
Marrowfat Peas, Mushy					
BATCHELORS	83		5.5	13.4	0.8
Chip Shop BATCHELORS	74		5	12.2	0.6
Mung Beans					
dried	279		23.9	46.3	1.1
dried, boiled	91		7.6	15.3	0.4
Pinto Beans					
canned	85		7	13	0.5
dried	327		21.1	57.1	1.6
dried, boiled	137		8.9	23.9	0.7
refried	107		6.2	15.3	1.1
Red Kidney Beans					
canned	100		6.9	17.8	0.6
dried, boiled	103		8.4	17.4	0.5
canned BATCHELORS	87		7.6	12.6	0.7

Food Type	cal per 100g	cal per portion	pro (g)	carb (g)	fat (g)
canned BONDUELLE	103		8.4	10.7	0.5
Refried Beans					
DISCOVERY FOODS	89		5.3	15.8	0.5
OLD EL PASO	93		6.1	16.1	0.4
spicy DISCOVERY FOODS	90		5.3	16	0.5
Soya Beans					
dried	370		35.9	15.8	18.6
dried, boiled	141		14	5.1	7.3
Split Peas					
dried, boiled	126		8.3	22.7	0.9
yellow, dried NATCO	343		22.1	58.2	2.4
Tofu (soya bean curd)					
steamed	73		8.1	0.7	4.2
steamed, fried	261		23.5	2	17.7
Baked Beans & Baked Bean Products					
Baked Beans					
in tomato sauce	84		5.2	15.3	0.6
Bloomin' Big, in tomato sauce					
BRANSTON	87		4.8	16.1	0.4
in tomato sauce BRANSTON	87		4.8	16.1	0.4
in tomato sauce HEINZ	72		4.6	12.9	0.2
in tomato sauce, no added sugar WEIGHTWATCHERS	66		4.7	11.3	0.2
in tomato sauce, organic HEINZ	72		4.7	12.8	0.2

Food Type	cal per 100g	cal per portion	pro (g)	carb (g)	fat (g)
in tomato sauce, reduced sugar & salt HEINZ	66		4.8	11.2	0.2
in tomato sauce, Snap Pots					
HEINZ	72		4.7	12.9	0.2
reduced sugar & salt BRANSTON	72		4.6	12.8	0.3
Baked Beans with Big Saucy Bangers					
HEINZ	104		5.7	11.9	3.7
Baked Beans with Pork Sausages					
HEINZ	93		5.3	10.6	3.3
Baked Beans with Red Hot Balls					
HEINZ	93		5.8	12.1	2.4
Baked Beans with Saucy Steak					
HEINZ	83		6.8	12.9	0.4
Baked Beans with Sausages					
BRANSTON	100		6.3	13.4	2.3
Baked Beans & Mini Sausages with Omega 3					
HEINZ	86		5.3	9.5	2.9
BBQ Beans					
HEINZ	82		4.9	14.9	0.3
Bolognese Beanfeast					
as served BATCHELORS		54	4.7	7	0.8
Chilli Beans in a Chilli Sauce					
canned, organic BIONA	78		5.4	12.5	0.5

Food Type	cal per 100g	cal per portion	pro (g)	carb (g)	fat (g)
Curry Beans					
HEINZ	96		4.8	16.3	1.3
Hunger Breaks					
All Day Breakfast HL FOODS	89		4.8	6.6	4
Big BBQ HL FOODS	107		6	8.9	5
Full Monty HL FOODS	81		5.6	7.2	3.8
Mean Beanz					
Mexican HEINZ	76		5	12.9	0.5
smoky barbecue HEINZ	79		4.8	14.3	0.2
sweet chilli HEINZ	73		4.5	13	0.3
Mexican Chilli Beanfeast					
as sold BATCHELORS	312		24.3	42.7	4.9
Cereal Products					
Barley, Pearl					
as sold	361		9.9	77.7	1.2
80g serving, cooked		101	1.8	22.6	0.4
Bran					
Oatbran Sprinkles MORNFLAKE	345		14.8	49.5	9.7
wheat	206		14.1	26.8	5.5
wheat JORDANS	204		14	24.5	5.5
Bulgar Wheat					
organic, as sold BIONA	338		12.6	73.4	2
Couscous					
as sold JULIAN GRAVES	364		13	74	1.8

Food Type	cal per 100g	cal per portion	pro (g)	carb (g)	fat (g)
Citrus Kick, per serving					
AINSLEY HARRIOTT		182	5.6	36.3	1.6
Moroccan Medley, per serving					
AINSLEY HARRIOTT		178	7	33	2
Premium, per serving					
AINSLEY HARRIOTT		153	6.6	29.6	0.9
Roasted Vegetable Style, per serving AINSLEY HARRIOTT		180	7.3	33.2	2
Spice Sensation, per serving					
AINSLEY HARRIOTT		165	5.6	31.1	2
Tomato Tango, per serving					
AINSLEY HARRIOTT		168	6	31.9	1.8
Wickedly Wild Mushroom, per serving AINSLEY HARRIOTT		193	8.4	38.6	1.4
Linseed					
as sold HOLLAND & BARRETT	348		21.8	0.7	32.7
Polenta					
ready-made ITALFRESCO		72	16	15.7	0.3
Quinoa					
organic, as sold BIOFAIR	374		13.1	71	5.8
flakes, organic, as sold BIOFAIR	399		13.8	72.2	5.7
Wheatgerm	357		26.7	44.7	9.2
JORDANS	362		28.4	41.4	9.2

Food Type	cal per 100g	cal per portion	pro (g)	carb (g)	fat (g)
Biscuits					
Sweet Biscuits					
Abernethy Biscuits					
SIMMERS	475		6.6	65.6	20.7
Arrowroot, Thin					
CRAWFORD'S	472		7.1	76.7	15.2
Boasters					
cranberry & almond MCVITIE'S	494		6.3	61.9	24.5
dark chocolate & ginger MCVITIE'S	490		5.5	63.7	23.7
Belgian chocolate chunk MCVITIE'S	504		5.5	59.5	27.1
Belgian chocolate chunk & hazelnut MCVITIE'S	530		6.9	52.8	32.4
Bourbon Creams					
LYONS	488		4.6	64.7	24.6
Caramel Digestive Shortcakes					
MCVITIE'S	478		5.6	65.1	21.7
Caramel Log					
TUNNOCK'S	468		4.2	65.7	21
Caramel Wafers					
TUNNOCK'S	448		3.6	69.2	17.4
WEIGHTWATCHERS	427		5.7	64.7	20.2
Dark Chocolate TUNNOCK'S	455		3.6	69.9	17.9
Chocolate Biscuit Cakes					
gluten-free GRANNY ANN	494		10.9	51.7	27.1

Food Type	cal per 100g	cal per portion	pro (g)	carb (g)	fat (g)
Chocolate Chip Cookies					
CADBURY	503		5.9	62.2	25.6
Double CADBURY	485		7.3	64.3	22.2
Double WEIGHTWATCHERS	445		4.7	69.7	16.4
Real WEIGHTWATCHERS	463		4.9	71.5	17.5
Chocolate Oliver Biscuits					
HUNTLEY & PALMER	515		4.8	61.1	30.2
Chocolate Viennese Melts					
FOX'S	540		6.4	57.2	31.7
MCVITIE'S	530		6	61	29.1
Chocolate Wafer Cream					
TUNNOCK'S	512		5.4	62.4	26.8
Cranberry & Orange Cookies					
WEIGHTWATCHERS	448		4.3	69.9	16.8
Chunkie Cookies					
dark chocolate chunk FOX'S	446		4.4	56.1	22.7
extremely chocolatey FOX'S	506		6.2	61	26.3
milk chocolate chunk FOX'S	502		6	61.8	25.7
white chocolate chunk FOX'S	505		5.8	62.8	25.7
Club Biscuits					
milk chocolate JACOB'S	506		5.4	61	26.7
Coconut Rings					
LYONS	493		6.9	62.7	23.8
Custard Creams					
LYONS	499		5.3	64.3	23.2

Food Type	cal per 100g	cal per portion	pro (g)	carb (g)	fat (g)
Digestive Biscuits					
chocolate (milk & dark)	493		6.8	66.5	24.1
Bournville CADBURY	490		6.8	61.6	23.9
Dark Chocolate MCVITIE'S	486		6	61.5	24
Milk Chocolate CADBURY	495		6.8	62.3	24.4
Milk Chocolate MCVITIE'S	488		6.7	62.7	23.4
Milk Chocolate, Light MCVITIE'S	450		7.2	69.6	15.8
Milk Chocolate, Mini MCVITIE'S	496		6.6	61.9	24.7
plain	465		6.3	68.6	20.3
Plain HOVIS	306		6.2	66.8	18.5
Plain MCVITIE'S	470		7.2	62.7	21.5
Plain, Light MCVITIE'S	445		7.1	67.9	16.1
Plain, Organic DOVES FARM	446		5.9	61.6	19.5
Double Chocolate Viennese Melts					
FOX'S	541		6.3	57	32
Echo Chocolate					
FOX'S	513		7.1	60.7	26.7
Echo Mint					
FOX'S	512		7.1	60.7	26.8
Favourites					
FOX'S	495		6.1	64.3	23.8
Figfuls					
Go ahead! MCVITIE'S	365		4.2	76.8	4.6

Food Type	cal per 100g	cal per portion	pro (g)	carb (g)	fat (g)
Fig Rolls					
JACOB'S	354		3.7	67.6	7.7
Fingers					
dark chocolate CADBURY	505		6.2	59	26.9
double chocolate CADBURY	515		6.9	60.2	27.1
milk chocolate CADBURY	515		6.8	60.8	27.1
white CADBURY	535		60.1	60.7	29.6
Fruit Crunch					
RYVITA	366		10.9	65.8	6.6
Fruit Shortcake					
MCVITIE'S	464		5.7	65.1	20.1
Fruit & Spice Oat Biscuits					
NAIRN	412		8.6	65.3	12.9
Fruity Oat Biscuits					
organic, DOVES FARM	453		7.5	65.1	18.1
Garibaldi	397		5.1	70.8	10.4
Ginger Crunch Creams					
FOX'S	503		4.7	65.4	24.8
Ginger & Lemon Cookies					
WEIGHTWATCHERS	451		4.2	70.6	16.9
Gingernut Biscuits	436		5.6	79.1	13
MCVITIE'S	456		5.8	70.9	16.5
Go ahead! Crispy Slice					
apple & sultana MCVITIE'S	385		5.7	73.1	7.7
chocolate MCVITIE'S	398		6.8	68.4	10.8

Food Type	cal per 100g	cal per portion	pro (g)	carb (g)	fat (g)
forest fruits MCVITIE'S	386		5.7	73.6	7.6
orange & sultana MCVITIE'S	386		5.7	73.6	7.6
Go ahead! Mallows					
MCVITIE'S	401		4.7	69.7	11.5
Go ahead! Yogurt Breaks					
blueberry MCVITIE'S	404		5.9	71.9	10.3
forest fruit MCVITIE'S	404		5.6	71.4	10.7
plain MCVITIE'S	400		6.6	69.2	10.8
raspberry MCVITIE'S	402		5.8	71.8	10.2
strawberry MCVITIE'S	396		5.9	68	11.1
tropical fruits MCVITIE'S	404		5.6	71.4	10.7
Golden Crunch Creams					
FOX'S	515		5	64.9	26.2
Hazelnut Cookies					
organic DOVES FARM	484		4.5	56.8	26.8
Hob Nobs					
MCVITIE'S	467		7.1	60.9	21.7
chocolate cream MCVITIE'S	498		5.9	56.8	27.4
light MCVITIE'S	428		8.1	65.5	14.8
milk chocolate MCVITIE'S	480		6.8	60.8	23.3
mini chocolate MCVITIE'S	483		6.7	61.1	23.6
plain chocolate MCVITIE'S	480		6.2	60.1	23.9
vanilla cream MCVITIE'S	480		6.2	60.1	23.9
Iced Gems					
JACOB'S	388		5	85.5	2.9

Biscuits

Food Type	cal per 100g	cal per portion	pro (g)	carb (g)	fat (g)
Jaffa Cakes					
CADBURY	375		5.1	66.1	9.9
MCVITIE'S	374		4.8	70.6	8.1
Jam Ring Creams					
FOX'S	497		6.1	64.8	23.7
Jammie Dodgers					
BURTON'S	437		5.1	69.5	15.9
berrilicious BURTON'S	436		5	67.7	15.8
jam 'n custard BURTON'S	438		5.1	68.3	16
mini BURTON'S	452		5.5	72.7	14.7
Knobbles					
oat & honey HUNTLEY & PALMER	520		4.6	65.2	27.8
oat & lemon HUNTLEY & PALMER	520		4.6	65.2	27.8
Lemon Puffs					
JACOB'S	543		5.9	62.8	29.8
Lemon Zest Cookies					
organic DOVES FARM	435		3.1	67.6	17.3
Mallos					
CADBURY	465		5.1	69.4	18.8
Maryland Chocolate Chip Cookies					
CADBURY	511		6.2	68	23.9
Maryland Chocolate Chip, Oatmeal & Honey Cookies					
CADBURY	512		6	66	25

Food Type	cal per 100g	cal per portion	pro (g)	carb (g)	fat (g)
Maryland Chocolate Chip & Hazelnut Cookies					
CADBURY	513		6.3	65.3	25
Millionaire's Shortcakes					
FOX'S	496		6	58.7	26.3
Mixed Berry Oat Biscuits					
NAIRN	430		7.7	67	14.6
Nice Biscuits	485		6.5	68	20.8
Nice Creams					
FOX'S	505		4.6	67.3	24
Nutri-Grain Soft Oaties					
oat & chocolate chip KELLOGG'S	452		6	62	20
oat & raisin KELLOGG'S	432		6	66	16
Oatflake & Cranberry Biscuits					
WALKERS	480		5.8	60.9	23.7
Orange Viennese Melts					
MCVITIE'S	525		6.4	59.5	29.1
Party Rings					
FOX'S	440		5	73.6	15
Penguin Biscuit					
MCVITIE'S	520		5.2	62.4	27.7
Penguin Wafer Bar					
MCVITIE'S	522		5.8	55.7	30.7
Raspberry & White Chocolate Cookies					
WEIGHTWATCHERS	443		5.2	71.4	17.2

Food Type	cal per 100g	cal per portion	pro (g)	carb (g)	fat (g)
Rich Tea Biscuits					
MCVITIE'S	453		7.1	71.2	15.5
Light MCVITIE'S	428		7.5	75.5	10.7
Milk Chocolate CADBURY	480		7.2	66.5	20.3
Rocky					
FOX'S	507		6.9	60.3	26.4
caramel FOX'S	480		5.9	62.2	23.1
orange FOX'S	513		7.1	43	26.7
Shortbread					
Dark Chocolate Rings WALKER'S	527		5.3	58.8	30.1
Fingers WALKER'S	531		4.4	59.9	30.4
Vanilla WALKER'S	556		4.9	59.5	32.9
Shortcake					
CADBURY	500		6.3	65.7	23.5
Espresso Chocolate MCVITIE'S	538		6.4	54.2	32.9
Fruit & Nut Caramel MCVITIE'S	482		5.3	60.4	24.4
Milk Chocolate FOX'S	520		8	58.7	27.8
Toffee Crunch MCVITIE'S	523		5.7	62.7	27.8
Snack					
Shortcake CADBURY	525		7	64.2	26.8
Snowballs					
TUNNOCK'S	446		4.2	56.7	20.8
Sports Biscuits					
FOX'S	483		6.7	67	20.9
Stem Ginger Biscuits					
WALKER'S	498		4.7	63	25.2

Food Type	cal per 100g	cal per portion	pro (g)	carb (g)	fat (g)
Stem Ginger Oat Biscuits					
NAIRN	434		8.3	66.6	14.9
Strawberry & Cream Cookies					
WEIGHTWATCHERS	441		4.2	70.9	15.6
Taxi					
MCVITIE'S	468		3.4	55.7	25.7
Tea Cakes					
TUNNOCK'S	440		4.9	61.9	19.2
dark chocolate TUNNOCK'S	436		4.2	61	19.5
Teacakes, Jam					
BURTON'S	455		3.8	66.9	19.3
Toffee Cookies					
WEIGHTWATCHERS	456		5.2	71.1	16.8
Toffeepops					
BURTON'S	470		4.9	67.2	20.3
Viennese Whirls					
MR KIPLING	517		4	56	30.8
Wafer Biscuits					
filled	537		4.7	66	30.1
Wagon Wheels					
chocolate BURTON'S	431		5.1	66.9	15.6
jammie BURTON'S	425		4.9	63.2	15
Whipped Creams					
lustful lemon FOX'S	553		5.5	51.9	36
sinfully strawberry FOX'S	551		5.5	52.4	35.6

Biscuits

Food Type	cal per 100g	cal per portion	pro (g)	carb (g)	fat (g)
White Chocolate Chunk & Raspberry Biscuits					
WALKERS	493		5.5	60.2	25.6
Winter Spice Cookies					
WEIGHTWATCHERS	443		2.5	72.2	16
Savoury Biscuits & Crispbreads					
Bath Oliver					
FORTTS	432		9.6	67.5	13.7
Cheddar Cheese Biscuits					
organic DOVES FARM	414		11	42.6	22.1
Cheddars					
JACOB'S	509		11.6	53.2	27.2
Cheese Melts					
CARR'S	481		12.1	57.4	22.5
Cheeselets					
JACOB'S	492		9.8	55.5	25.7
Choice Grain Cracker					
JACOB'S	429		9.1	66	14.3
Cornish Wafers					
JACOB'S	528		8.3	53.3	31.3
Crackerbread					
RYVITA	380		10.3	76.9	3.5
wholegrain RYVITA	360		12.4	68.7	3.9

Food Type	cal per 100g	cal per portion	pro (g)	carb (g)	fat (g)
Cream Crackers					
standard	414		9.5	68.3	13.3
JACOB'S	431		10	67.6	13.5
high fibre JACOB'S	452		9.2	59.5	19.6
light JACOB'S	388		10.7	72.5	6.1
roasted garlic JACOB'S	434		9.8	66.9	14.2
Croutons					
Garlic & Herb SOUP SHOT	434		13.2	63.8	14
Lightly Salted RAIN TREE	434		9.2	72.8	11.7
Sea Salt SOUP SHOT	452		12	61.1	17.8
Croutons, Salad					
Mediterranean LA ROCHELLE	510		25	8.5	12.5
Hovis Cracker					
JACOB'S	447		10.2	60	18.5
Hovis Digestive for Cheese					
JACOB'S	468		7.5	64.8	19.9
Krackawheat					
MCVITIE'S	446		9.6	60.5	18.5
Melts					
CARR'S	465		11	57.6	21
Oat Cracker					
JACOB'S	443		14.4	59.2	16.5
PATERSON'S	431		10.7	58.5	17.1
Oat Crunch Biscuits					
WEIGHTWATCHERS	446		7.1	63.7	18

Food Type	cal per 100g	cal per portion	pro (g)	carb (g)	fat (g)
Oatcakes					
Black Pepper PATERSON'S	430		10.6	58.4	17.1
Bran PATERSON'S	416		10	58.4	15.8
Cheesey NAIRN	476		13.3	45.5	26.7
Fine NAIRN	448		10.8	53.7	21.1
Herb NAIRN	462		13.9	45	25.2
Mini NAIRN	448		10.8	53.7	21.1
Olive Oil PATERSON'S	430		10.6	58.3	17.2
Organic NAIRN	399		12.5	51.6	15.8
Rough NAIRN	419		11.2	53.2	17.9
Rough PATERSON'S	430		10.6	58.3	17.2
Scottish PATERSON'S	430		10.6	58.3	17.2
Triangle PATERSON'S	431		10.6	58.1	17.3
Ritz Crackers					
JACOB'S	493		7	57.5	26.1
cheese JACOB'S	481		8.9	56.6	24.4
Rosemary & Thyme Savoury Biscuits					
WEIGHTWATCHERS	414		7.7	51.9	19.5
Rye Crispbread	308		9.4	70.6	0.6
Ryvita					
RYVITA	317		8.5	66.6	1.7
dark rye RYVITA	336		10.5	58.8	6.5
garlic & rosemary RYVITA	327		8.4	70.1	1.4
multigrain RYVITA	331		10	61.1	5.2

Food Type	cal per 100g	cal per portion	pro (g)	carb (g)	fat (g)
pumpkin seeds & oats RYVITA	362		12.5	55.6	1.3
sesame RYVITA	336		10.5	58.8	6.5
sunflower seeds & oats RYVITA	348		10.1	57.2	8.8
tomato & basil RYVITA	316		8.7	66.2	1.8
Savours					
garlic & herb JACOB'S	446		9.1	65.6	16.3
rosemary & sea salt JACOB'S	477		7.8	62.7	21.7
salt & cracked black pepper JACOB'S	453		9.1	67	16.5
sesame & roasted onion JACOB'S	489		8.7	59.9	23.8
Sun-Dried Tomato & Italian Herb Savoury Biscuits					
WEIGHTWATCHERS	417		8	51.7	19.8
Thins					
cracked black pepper RYVITA	402		14	69.6	7.5
multi-seed RYVITA	385		16	60	9
Tuc Biscuits					
JACOB'S	522		7	60.5	28
Tuc Cheese Sandwich Biscuits					
JACOB'S	531		8.4	53.8	31.4
Water Biscuits					
High Bake JACOB'S	412		11	75.6	7.3
Table CARR'S	406		10.1	74.2	7.6
Wholemeal Crackers	413		10.1	72.1	11.3

Food Type	cal per 100g	cal per portion	pro (g)	carb (g)	fat (g)
Breakfast Cereals					
Breakfast Cereals					
3 in One					
raisins & apple JORDANS	340		7.6	67.4	4.4
strawberries JORDANS	362		9.4	68	5.8
All-Bran					
KELLOGG'S	280		14	48	3.5
Bran Flakes					
KELLOGG'S	326		10	67	2
Sultana Bran KELLOGG'S	318		8	67	2
Cheerios					
NESTLÉ	385		9.3	74.5	5.6
honey NESTLÉ	369		6.6	79.2	2.8
Clusters					
NESTLÉ	371		9.3	72.6	4.8
Coco Pops					
KELLOGG'S	387		5	85	3
Cookie Crisp					
NESTLÉ	375		6.4	80.4	3.1
Corn Flakes					
KELLOGG'S	372		7	84	0.9
Multi-Grain KELLOGG'S	370		8	81	1.5
Organic DOVES FARM	378		10.3	81.7	1
With a Hint of Honey KELLOGG'S	377		6	87	0.6

Food Type	cal per 100g	cal per portion	pro (g)	carb (g)	fat (g)
Crunchy Bran					
WEETABIX	306		11.9	56.6	3.6
Crunchy Nut Bites					
KELLOGG'S	438		6	70	15
Crunchy Nut Clusters					
honey & nut KELLOGG'S	439		8	68	15
milk chocolate curls KELLOGG'S	458		8	66	18
summer berries KELLOGG'S	439		8	68	15
Crunchy Nut Cornflakes					
KELLOGG'S	397		6	82	5
nutty KELLOGG'S	418		7	75	10
Crunchy Oat Bakes, All-Bran					
KELLOGG'S	395		7	58	15
Curiously Cinnamon					
NESTLÉ	412		4.9	75.9	9.9
Fitnesse					
NESTLÉ	363		8	79.8	1.3
and fruit NESTLÉ	351		8.8	67.2	5.2
honey & nut NESTLÉ	376		7.2	80.2	2.9
Flakes & Berries					
organic JORDANS	358		8.5	74.7	2.8
Force					
NESTLÉ	342		10.6	70.6	1.9
Frosted Wheats					
KELLOGG'S	346		10	72	2

Food Type	cal per 100g	cal per portion	pro (g)	carb (g)	fat (g)
Frosties					
KELLOGG'S	371		4.5	87	0.6
Fruit 'n' Fibre					
KELLOGG'S	358		8	68	6
Fruit & Fibre Flakes					
organic JORDANS	364		9.9	66	6.7
Golden Nuggets					
NESTLÉ	378		6.9	84.2	1.5
Grape Nuts					
KRAFT	345		11.5	70	2
Honey Loops					
KELLOGG'S	363		8	76	3
Honey Waffles					
HONEY MONSTER FOODS	373		6.5	77	4.4
Just Right					
KELLOGG'S	366		7	80	2
Multi-Grain Start					
KELLOGG'S	378		8	79	3.5
Naturally Light Flakes					
with cranberries, cherries & raspberries DORSET CEREALS	330		10.2	58.7	6
with figs & grapes DORSET CEREALS	342		9.9	72.3	1.5
with pomegranate & cherries DORSET CEREALS	343		9.6	72	1.8

Food Type	cal per 100g	cal per portion	pro (g)	carb (g)	fat (g)
Nesquik Breakfast Cereal					
NESTLÉ	379		7.3	79.1	3.8
Oat Crisp					
QUAKER	364		10.5	60.8	6.8
Oatbran Flakes					
MORNFLAKE	354		10.4	65.8	5.4
very berry MORNFLAKE	351		11.4	66.3	4.5
Oatibix					
WEETABIX	377		12.5	63.7	8
Oatibix Bites					
WEETABIX	370		10.6	66.5	6.8
with chocolate & raisin					
WEETABIX	389		10.3	64.4	10
Oatibix Flakes					
WEETABIX	381		9.5	73.2	5.6
with raisin, cranberry &					
blackcurrant WEETABIX	363		7.5	74.1	4.2
Oats & More					
almond NESTLÉ	398		10.7	68.7	8.9
honey NESTLÉ	379		9.7	73.1	5.3
raisin NESTLÉ	373		8.9	73.7	4.7
Puffed Wheat					
HONEY MONSTER FOODS	365		11.5	74	2.5
Raisin Wheats					
KELLOGG'S	327		9	69	2

Breakfast Cereals

Food Type	cal per 100g	cal per portion	pro (g)	carb (g)	fat (g)
Rice Krispies					
KELLOGG'S	381		6	87	1
multi-grain shapes KELLOGG'S	370		8	77	2.5
Ricicles					
KELLOGG'S	381		4.5	89	0.8
Shredded Wheat					
NESTLÉ	340		11.6	67.8	2.5
bitesize NESTLÉ	350		11.8	69.9	2.6
fruitful NESTLÉ	351		8.8	67.2	5.2
honey nut NESTLÉ	378		11.2	68.8	6.5
Shreddies					
coco NESTLÉ	358		8.5	76.6	2
frosted NESTLÉ	358		8.3	77.7	1.6
honey NESTLÉ	359		8.2	78.1	1.5
Special K					
KELLOGG'S	374		15	75	1.5
medley KELLOGG'S	363		7	78	2.5
oats & honey KELLOGG'S	383		13	77	2.5
peach & apricot KELLOGG'S	378		14	77	1.5
purple berries KELLOGG'S	374		13	77	1.5
red berries KELLOGG'S	374		14	76	1.5
yoghurty KELLOGG'S	383		14	75	3
Special K Bliss					
creamy berry crunch KELLOGG'S	383		13	76	3
strawberry & chocolate KELLOGG'S	383		13	76	3

Food Type	cal per 100g	cal per portion	pro (g)	carb (g)	fat (g)
Sugar Puffs					
HONEY MONSTER FOODS	379		5.3	85.8	1.6
Superfoods Breakfast Flakes					
JORDANS	349		9.2	68.1	4.4
Sustain					
KELLOGG'S	338		14	66	2
Weetabix					
WEETABIX	338		11.5	68.4	2
bitesize WEETABIX	338		11.5	68.4	2
organic WEETABIX	338		11.5	68.4	2
Weetos					
chocolate flavour WEETABIX	377		8.4	74.7	4.9
Weetaflakes					
WEETABIX	353		9	76.4	1.3
with raisin, cranberry &					
apple WEETABIX	354		7	77.4	1.8
Hot Cereals					
Fruity Porridge					
apple & raisin, as sold					
DORSET CEREALS	333		9.7	62.7	4.8
cranberry & raspberry, as sold					
DORSET CEREALS	330		10.2	58.7	6
date & banana, as sold					
DORSET CEREALS	333		10	59.4	6.1

Food Type	cal per 100g	cal per portion	pro (g)	carb (g)	fat (g)
Honey Meltz					
HONEY MONSTER FOODS	379		8.3	70	9.5
Lyle's Golden Syrup Porridge Oats					
MORNFLAKE	365		6.8	73.4	4.9
Oatmeal					
Medium HAMLYNS	392		11	60	8
Oats					
Jumbo MORNFLAKE	356		11	60	8
Maple Flavour Real Fruit & Nut Porridge QUAKER	330		8.5	55	8.5
Organic JORDANS	364		11.7	58.4	9.3
Organic MORNFLAKE	356		11	60	8
Organic QUAKER	356		11	60	8
Porridge JORDANS	364		11.7	58.4	9.3
Quaker QUAKER	356		11	60	8
Real Fruit Porridge QUAKER	320		8.5	59	5.5
Scott's Porage QUAKER	356		11	60	8
Superfast MORNFLAKE	356		11	60	8
Superfast with 20% wheat bran MORNFLAKE	320		11.4	52.3	7.2
Oats 2 Go					
MORNFLAKE	359		11	60.4	8.1
Oatso Simple					
QUAKER	364		11	60	8.5

Food Type	cal per 100g	cal per portion	pro (g)	carb (g)	fat (g)
apple & blueberry QUAKER	364		8.4	68	6.3
golden syrup QUAKER	366		8.4	68.7	6.2
maple flavoured fruit &					
nut QUAKER	360		9	58.5	10.5
nuts, seeds & orchard fruits					
QUAKER	365		10	57.5	11
raspberry QUAKER	364		8.8	67.1	6.5
sultana, raisins, cranberry &					
apple QUAKER	348		8	66.1	5.8
Porridge					
made with water		46	1.4	8.1	1.1
made with whole milk		113	4.8	12.6	5.1
Porridge, Perfectly					
as sold DORSET CEREALS	356		11.8	58.2	8.4
Ready Brek					
WEETABIX	359		11.8	58.5	8.7
chocolate WEETABIX	361		9.9	64.2	7.2
Scott's So-Easy					
QUAKER	364		11	60	8.5
Muesli & Granola					
Alpen					
WEETABIX	357		11	66.9	5
high fibre WEETABIX	343		7.7	62.1	7.1
high fruit WEETABIX	170		4	34.4	1.8
no added sugar WEETABIX	141		4.4	26	2.1

Food Type	cal per 100g	cal per portion	pro (g)	carb (g)	fat (g)
Classic Oat Crunchy					
MORNFLAKE	400		8	63	12.9
Country Crisp					
flame raisin JORDANS	407		6.5	66.3	12.9
four nut JORDANS	481		9	55.7	24.7
honey clusters JORDANS	433		7.7	67.1	14.9
raspberry JORDANS	435		7.7	65.3	15.9
strawberry JORDANS	435		7.7	65.3	15.9
Country Store					
KELLOGG'S	353		9	68	5
Crunchy Oats					
with raisins, almonds &					
honey JORDANS	409		8.7	64.3	13
with special fruits & nuts JORDANS	409		7.6	64.2	13.5
with tropical fruits JORDANS	423		8.6	65.5	14.1
Extra Crispy Muesli					
4-nut favourite MORNFLAKE	399		13	47.1	17.6
5-fruit, nut & seeds MORNFLAKE	363		10.3	57.2	10.3
date, fig & apple MORNFLAKE	381		10.7	54.3	13.4
Swiss-style with apple MORNFLAKE	367		10.8	59	9.7
Granny Smith Apple Oat					
Crisp Cereal					
MORNFLAKE	398		7.3	63.3	10.6
Granola					
organic JORDANS	428		9.1	62.5	15.7

Food Type	cal per 100g	cal per portion	pro (g)	carb (g)	fat (g)
Hawaiian Oat Crunch					
MORNFLAKE	418		6	69.3	13
Honey Granola					
DORSET CEREALS	484		12.6	51.2	25.4
Minis					
chocolate crisp WEETABIX	371		9	71.7	5.3
fruit & nut crisp WEETABIX	359		9.3	70	4.6
honey & nut crisp WEETABIX	368		9.9	70.6	5.1
Muesli					
Swiss style	362		9	68	6
Swiss style with no added sugar or salt	358		10	66	6
Berries & Cherries DORSET CEREALS	321		6.5	68.8	2.2
Exotic Fruit QUAKER	365		10	61	9.5
Fruit, Nuts & Seeds DORSET CEREALS	379		10.6	58.4	11.4
Fruit, Nuts & Seeds, Organic DORSET CEREALS	358		10.8	56.6	9.8
Fruit & Nut JORDANS	361		8	61.2	9.4
Fruit & Nut QUAKER	345		9.5	65	5
Fruity Fibre JORDANS	344		7.6	64.3	6.3
Harvest Fruit QUAKER	360		8.5	63	8.5
High Fibre JULIAN GRAVES	348		9.8	71	2.8
Luxury KELLOGG'S	358		9	58	10
Natural JORDANS	327		8.7	61.2	5.3
Nut & Seed JORDANS	398		11.1	53.1	15.7

Food Type	cal per 100g	cal per portion	pro (g)	carb (g)	fat (g)
Organic JORDANS	350		9.3	58.4	8.8
Really Nutty DORSET CEREALS	362		9.8	61.1	8.7
Simply Delicious DORSET CEREALS	366		10.8	59.2	9.5
Super Berry JORDANS	348		9	60.8	7.6
Super Cranberry, Cherry & Almond DORSET CEREALS	365		9.6	62.9	7.9
Super High Fibre DORSET CEREALS	357		8	60.1	9.4
Tasty, Toasted Spelt, Barley & Oat Flakes DORSET CEREALS	371		9.5	57.9	11.3
Tropical JORDANS	329		6.9	68.7	2.9
Nature's Pleasure					
almonds, pecan & cashews KELLOGG'S	418		11	62	14
almonds, pecan & raisins KELLOGG'S	408		10	65	12
apple & blackcurrant KELLOGG'S	409		9	64	13
cherry & raspberry KELLOGG'S	414		9	63	14
Oat Granola					
QUAKER	411		8.6	73	8.8
with blackberries & red skin apple QUAKER	395		10	67	9.5
with strawberries & raspberries QUAKER	405		10	68	10
Optiva					
berry oat crisp KELLOGG'S	357		10	68	5

Food Type	cal per 100g	cal per portion	pro (g)	carb (g)	fat (g)
nut oat crisp KELLOGG'S	400		11	62	12
raisin oat crisp KELLOGG'S	341		9	68	4.5
Orchard Oat Crunchy					
MORNFLAKE	425		7.8	65.8	14.5
Superfoods Granola					
JORDANS	423		9.2	65.9	13.6
Cereal Bars					
Absolute Nut Luxury Bar					
each (45g) JORDANS		250	5.7	15	18.6
All-Bran Honey & Oat Bar					
KELLOGG'S	366		6	67	8
Almond, Cherry & Apricot Cereal Bar					
organic, each (50g) GREEN & BLACK		229	3.9	26.7	11.8
Alpen Apple & Blackberry Cereal Bar, with yoghurt					
each WEETABIX		117	1.6	20.8	3.1
Alpen Fruit & Nut Cereal Bar					
each (28g) WEETABIX		109	2	20.4	2.2
Alpen Fruit & Nut Cereal Bar with chocolate					
each (29g) WEETABIX		125	2.1	20.2	3.9

Food Type	cal per 100g	cal per portion	pro (g)	carb (g)	fat (g)
Alpen Groove Nutty Chocolate Bar					
each (32g) WEETABIX		140	2.4	21.4	5
Alpen Light Apple & Sultana Bar					
each (21g) WEETABIX		59	1.2	11.8	0.8
Alpen Light Chocolate & Fudge Bar					
each (21g) WEETABIX		62	1.2	11.4	1.3
Alpen Light Chocolate & Orange Bar					
each (21g) WEETABIX		60	1.3	11.5	1
Alpen Light Summer Fruits Bar					
each (21g) WEETABIX		59	1.2	11.9	0.8
Alpen Raspberry Cereal Bar, with yoghurt					
each (29g) WEETABIX		120	1.6	21.8	3
Alpen Strawberry Cereal Bar, with yoghurt					
each (29g) WEETABIX		121	1.7	21.5	3.1
Apple Crunch Crunchy Granola Bar					
per portion (42g) NATURE VALLEY		185	3.1	29	6.3
Apple & Sultana Cereal Bar					
organic, each (36g) SEEDS OF CHANGE		128	1.7	25.5	2.1

Food Type	cal per 100g	cal per portion	pro (g)	carb (g)	fat (g)
Berries & Cherries Bar					
each (35g) DORSET CEREALS		127	2	25.9	1.7
Breakfast-in-a-Bar					
cranberry & raspberry, each					
(40g) JORDANS		142	1.7	27.9	2.6
fruit & nut, each (40g) JORDANS		157	2.7	24.6	5.3
maple & pecan, each (40g)					
JORDANS		152	2.3	27.2	3.8
special muesli, each (40g)					
JORDANS		151	2.2	27	3.8
Brunch Bar					
cranberry & orange, each					
(35g) CADBURY		150	2.1	23.6	5.5
hazelnut, each (35g) CADBURY		160	2.4	21.2	7.5
raisin, each (35g) CADBURY		150	2	23.2	5.4
Canadian Maple Syrup Crunchy					
Granola Bar					
per portion (42g) NATURE VALLEY		179	3.4	27.4	6.9
Cereal & Milk Bar					
Coco Pops, each (20g) KELLOGG'S		85	1.5	14	2.5
Frosties, each (25g) KELLOGG'S		103	2	18	3
Rice Krispies, each (20g)					
KELLOGG'S		84	1.5	14	2.5
Chocolate & Crispy Rice Bar					
organic, each (35g) DOVES FARM		147	1.5	23.4	5.3

Food Type	cal per 100g	cal per portion	pro (g)	carb (g)	fat (g)
Chocolate & Raisin Cereal Bar,					
organic, each (29g) SEEDS OF CHANGE		107	1.5	20.2	2.3
Chunky Slice					
cranberry & almond, each					
(50g) DORSET CEREALS		193	3.4	31.7	5.8
date & pecan, each (50g)					
DORSET CEREALS		228	3.6	23.1	13.5
pistaschio & pumpkin seed,					
each (50g) DORSET CEREALS		210	4.7	28.6	8.6
Crunchy Bar					
honey & almond, each (30g)					
JORDANS		139	2.5	17	6.8
Crunchy Nut Caramely Peanut					
Crisp Bar					
each (35g) KELLOGG'S		167	4	19	8
Crunchy Nut Chocolatey Peanut					
Crisp Bar *each (35g)* KELLOGG'S		166	4	19	9
Crunchy Nut Nuts about					
Nuts Bar					
each (40g) KELLOGG'S		212	6	16	14
Crunchy Nut Nuts about					
Nuts 'n Fruit Bar					
KELLOGG'S	448		12	55	20
Fitnesse Bar					
chocolate, each NESTLÉ		90	1.2	17.6	1.6

Food Type	cal per 100g	cal per portion	pro (g)	carb (g)	fat (g)
chocolate & orange, each					
NESTLÉ		89	1.1	18.2	1.2
chocolate & raspberry, each					
NESTLÉ		88	1.1	17.9	1.4
multigrain, each NESTLÉ		90	1.3	17.6	1.6
strawberry, each NESTLÉ		90	1.2	17.6	1.6
Fruit & Fibre Cereal Bake					
KELLOGG'S	365		4.5	58	13
Fruit & Fibre Cereal Bar *each*					
(25g) KELLOGG'S		95	1.5	18	2.5
Fruits, Nuts & Seeds Bar					
each (35g) DORSET CEREALS		136	2.6	23.3	3.6
Fruity Oat Cereal Bar, *low-fat*					
organic, each (40g) DOVES FARM		142	2	28.6	1.1
Frusli Bar					
blueberry, each (30g) JORDANS		117	1.7	21.3	2.9
cranberry & apple, each (30g)					
JORDANS		117	1.7	21	3
raisin & hazelnut, each (30g)					
JORDANS		122	1.9	19.2	4.2
wild berries, each (30g) JORDANS		118	1.7	21.1	3
Go ahead! Bakes					
apple, each (35g) MCVITIE'S		124	0.9	25.8	2.5
blackberry & apple, each (35g)					
MCVITIE'S		124	0.9	25.8	2.5

Food Type	cal per 100g	cal per portion	pro (g)	carb (g)	fat (g)
raspberry, each (35g) MCVITIE'S		124	0.9	25.8	2.5
strawberry, each (35g) MCVITIE'S		124	0.9	25.9	2.5
strawberry twist, wholemeal, each MCVITIE'S		119	1.2	24.1	2.6
Go ahead! Cereal Bar					
almond, raisin & cranberry, each (35g) MCVITIE'S		117	2	19.6	3.4
apple & sultana, each (30g) MCVITIE'S		137	1.5	27.1	2.5
chocolate caramel crunch, each MCVITIE'S		106	1.1	17.8	3.4
hazelnut & pistachio, each (35g) MCVITIE'S		147	2	23.7	4.9
mixed berries, each MCVITIE'S		134	1.6	27	2.2
Goodness Bar					
luxury cranberry, date & almond, each (35g) RYVITA		111	2.2	20.8	2.1
luxury fruit & nut, each (35g) RYVITA		111	1.5	21.3	2.2
mixed berry, each (35g) RYVITA		61	1.2	12.6	0.7
Harvest Chewee					
milk chocolate chip, each (22g) HONEY MONSTER FOODS		92	1.1	15	3.2
white chocolate chip, each (22g) HONEY MONSTER FOODS		91	1.2	14.7	3.1

Food Type	cal per 100g	cal per portion	pro (g)	carb (g)	fat (g)
Lunchbox Bars					
Cheerios, each NESTLÉ		91	1.5	14.7	3
Honey Nut Cheerios, each NESTLÉ		89	1.4	14.7	2.7
Nesquik, each NESTLÉ		104	1.8	16.6	3.4
Nutri-grain Bar					
apple, each (37g) KELLOGG'S		131	1.5	24	3.5
blackberry & apple, each (37g)					
KELLOGG'S		131	1.5	25	3.5
blueberry, each (37g) KELLOGG'S		130	1.5	24	3.5
raspberry, each (37g) KELLOGG'S		131	1.5	25	3.5
strawberry, each (37g) KELLOGG'S		131	1.5	25	3.5
Nutri-grain Bar Elevenses					
carrot cake KELLOGG'S	375		4.5	67	10
chocolate chip, each (45g)					
KELLOGG'S		179	2	30	6
ginger, each (45g) KELLOGG'S		164	2.5	30	4
raisin, each (45g) KELLOGG'S		164	2.5	30	4
Nutri-grain Oat Baked Bars					
cherry, each (50g) KELLOGG'S		205	2.5	32	8
chocolate, each (50g) KELLOGG'S		204	2.5	31	8
totally oaty, each (50g)					
KELLOGG'S		206	2.5	32	8
Oat Bars					
each (38g) QUAKER		139	2.7	24.5	3.6

Food Type	cal per 100g	cal per portion	pro (g)	carb (g)	fat (g)
cranberry & blueberry, each					
(38g) QUAKER		137	2.6	24.5	3.3
Oats 'n Honey Crunchy					
Granola Bar					
per portion (42g) NATURE VALLEY		187	3.5	29.6	6.8
Oats & More Bar					
cherry, each (30g) NESTLÉ		109	1.8	21	2
chocolate, each (30g) NESTLÉ		118	2	20.5	3.1
strawberry, each (30g) NESTLÉ		109	1.8	21	2
Pecan, Hazelnut, Almond &					
Pumpkin Seed Cereal Bar					
organic, each (50g) GREEN & BLACK		258	4.2	23.6	16.3
Rice Krispies Squares					
each (28g) KELLOGG'S		118	0.8	21	3.5
chocolate & caramel, each					
(36g) KELLOGG'S		151	1.5	27	4.5
crazy choc, each (28g) KELLOGG'S		118	0.8	21	3.5
totally chocolatey, each					
(36g) KELLOGG'S		158	1.5	26	5
Special K Cereal Bar					
each (23g) KELLOGG'S		90	2	17	2
apple & pear, each (23g)					
KELLOGG'S		90	2	17	2
fruits of the forest, each (22g)					
KELLOGG'S		87	2	16	2

Food Type	cal per 100g	cal per portion	pro (g)	carb (g)	fat (g)
peach & apricot, each (23g)					
KELLOGG'S		90	2	17	2
Special K Mini Breaks					
per bag (24g) KELLOGG'S		98	2	17	2
lemon, per bag (24g) KELLOGG'S		98	2	17	2
Strawberry Cereal Bar					
organic, each (29g) SEEDS					
OF CHANGE		96	1.3	18.6	1.8
Super High Fibre Bar					
each (35g) DORSET CEREALS		149	3.4	21.2	5.6
Tracker Bar					
chocolate chip, each (26g) MARS		125	1.8	15.1	6.1
forest fruits MARS	448		4.4	63	18.6
raisin, each (26g) MARS		110	1.1	16.6	4.1
roasted nut, each (26g) MARS		127	2.1	14.3	6.6
Tropical Fruit & Nut Cereal Bar					
organic, each (40g) DOVES FARM		196	2.6	25.3	4.6
Weetos Cereal Bars					
each (20g) WEETABIX		88	1.2	14.2	2.9

Food Type	cal per 100g	cal per portion	pro (g)	carb (g)	fat (g)
Condiments & Sauces					
Table Sauces					
Balsamic & Mint Sauce					
organic BAXTERS	72		1.5	15.7	0.4
Bramley Apple Sauce					
BAXTERS	100		0.1	21.9	Tr
COLMAN'S	107		0.2	26.5	Tr
Barbecue Sauce, bottled					
classic HP	143		0.8	33.1	0.2
honey woodsmoke HP	126		0.6	32.2	0.2
hot 'n' sizzly HEINZ	132		1.1	31.2	0.3
spicy HP	156		0.9	36.7	0.1
Beetroot in Redcurrant Jelly					
BAXTERS	167		0.6	41	Tr
Brown Sauce					
bottled	98		1.2	22.2	0.1
BRANSTON	132		0.9	31.8	0.1
DADDIES	102		0.9	24.3	Tr
HP	119		1.1	27.1	0.2
Cranberry Jellied Sauce					
OCEAN SPRAY	156		0.2	38	0.3
Cranberry Jelly					
BAXTERS	268		Tr	67	Tr
Cranberry Sauce					
BAXTERS	180		0.1	45	0

Food Type	cal per 100g	cal per portion	pro (g)	carb (g)	fat (g)
extra fruit OCEAN SPRAY	205		0.3	50	0.4
organic OCEAN SPRAY	205		0.3	50	0.4
organic, wild ENGLISH PROVENDER CO.	274		0.3	67.3	0.4
smooth OCEAN SPRAY	156		0.2	38	0.3
whole berry OCEAN SPRAY	156		0.2	38	0.3
with mulled wine OCEAN SPRAY	225		0.3	55	0.4
Fruity Sauce					
HP	141		1.2	33.7	0.1
Horseradish Sauce					
BAXTERS	153		2.5	17.9	8.4
COLMAN'S	342		2.1	10.2	32.5
Hot ENGLISH PROVENDER CO.	112		1.9	9.8	6.2
Organic BAXTERS	157		1.8	19.5	8
	334		1.3	14.2	30.2
Japanese Soy Sauce					
BLUE DRAGON	63		8	8	0
Love Apple Tomato Sauce					
LEVI ROOTS	118		1.3	28	0.1
Mint Jelly					
BAXTERS	264		Tr	66	0
Mint Sauce					
BAXTERS	90		1.7	20	0.3
OAK LANE	115		1.5	26.4	0.3
Classic COLMAN'S	116		1	25.6	0.2
Fresh Garden COLMAN'S	116		1	25.6	0.2

Food Type

Food Type	cal per 100g	cal per portion	pro (g)	carb (g)	fat (g)
Mint Raita					
Meena's PATAK	84		3.2	7.8	4.8
Mushroom Ketchup					
GEO WATKINS	27		0.5	5.5	0.1
Oyster Sauce					
BLUE DRAGON	121		3.4	26.9	Tr
Peri-Peri Sauce					
extra hot NANDO'S	56		Tr	5.6	3.8
hot NANDO'S	65		Tr	5.2	4.8
medium NANDO'S	76		Tr	6.8	5.3
Redcurrant Jelly					
BAXTERS	260		0	65	0
Reggae Reggae Sauce					
LEVI ROOTS	121		1.1	28.8	0.1
Shoyu Soy Sauce					
MERIDIAN FOODS	67		8	8.4	0.3
Soy Sauce (light & dark)	43		3	8.2	Tr
Soy Sauce					
Chilli AMOY	55		4.6	9.1	0
Light SHARWOOD'S	37		2.7	6.4	0.2
Reduced Salt AMOY	56		4	10	0
Rich SHARWOOD'S	79		3.1	16.6	0.4
Steak Sauce					
HP	156		0.9	36.8	Tr

Food Type	cal per 100g	cal per portion	pro (g)	carb (g)	fat (g)
Sweet Chilli Sauce					
BLUE DRAGON	247		1.4	59.1	0.6
Tabasco Sauce					
per serving (1 tsp) TABASCO		0	0	0	0
Tartare Sauce					
BAXTERS	517		0.9	8.6	53.2
COLMAN'S	284		1.2	17	23
Organic BAXTERS	447		0.9	15.6	42.2
Tomato Ketchup	115		1.6	28.6	0.1
BRANSTON	116		1	27.9	0.1
DADDIES	110		0.9	26.5	Tr
HEINZ	102		0.9	23.9	0.1
Organic HEINZ	113		1.3	25.7	0.2
Organic MERIDIAN FOODS	112		1.7	25.3	Tr
Reduced Sugar & Salt HEINZ	71		1.1	15.1	0.1
With a Twist Chilli HEINZ	105		1	24.1	0.1
With a Twist Garlic HEINZ	97		1.1	22.2	0.1
With a Twist Sweet & Onion					
HEINZ	98		1.1	22.3	0.1
Tomato & Worcestershire Sauce					
LEA & PERRINS	102		0.8	23	0.5
Worcestershire Sauce					
LEA & PERRINS	92		0.9	22.2	0.1

Food Type

	cal per 100g	cal per portion	pro (g)	carb (g)	fat (g)
Mustards					
Dijon Mustard					
COLMAN'S	101		5.6	2.3	7.8
Original MAILLE	151		7	6	11
English Mustard					
prepared COLMAN'S	175		7	16.7	8.9
English Mustard Powder					
as sold COLMAN'S	516		32.3	10.6	32.2
Mild American Mustard					
COLMAN'S	92		4.7	8.3	4.5
Mild English Mustard					
COLMAN'S	84		5.3	5.4	4.6
Wholegrain Mustard					
COLMAN'S	154		8.8	8.9	9.3
Vinegars					
Balsamic Vinegar					
CARLO MAGNO	54		0.1	12.5	0
Organic ASPALL	89		0.5	17.5	0
Cider Vinegar					
ASPALL	18		0	0.1	0
Cyder Vinegar					
organic ASPALL	18		0	0.4	0
Malt Vinegar	20		0.3	0.4	0.1
Red Wine Vinegar					
ASPALL	22		0.6	0.4	0

Food Type	cal per 100g	cal per portion	pro (g)	carb (g)	fat (g)
Rice Vinegar					
BLUE DRAGON	6		0.2	1.4	0
MITSUKAN	26		0.2	2.6	0
White Wine Vinegar					
ASPALL	22		0	0.6	0
Stock Cubes, Granules & Purées					
Aromat					
KNORR	126		12.9	11.2	3.3
Beef Gravy Mix					
sachet COLMAN'S	318		15.8	59.1	2
sachet OXO	318		7.1	49.8	10
Beef Gravy Granules					
winter berry & shallot flavour, as prepared OXO		23	0.6	4.3	0.3
Beef Stock Cubes					
prepared (100ml) BOVRIL		7	0.5	0.9	0.1
prepared (100ml) KNORR		7	0.1	0.4	0.5
prepared (100ml) OXO		9	0.6	1.3	0.2
Bisto Favourite Gravy Granules					
as sold BISTO	398		2.2	60.7	16.3
reduced salt, as sold BISTO	413		2.6	64	16.3
Bisto Original Gravy Powder					
as sold BISTO	257		2.1	61.9	0.1

Food Type	cal per 100g	cal per portion	pro (g)	carb (g)	fat (g)
Chestnut Purée					
MERCHANT GOURMET	133		1.5	27.1	2
Chicken Granulated Stock					
as sold KNORR	232		13.1	36.5	3.7
Chicken Gravy Granules					
as sold BISTO	400		1.9	62.5	15.8
Chicken Gravy Mix					
sachet COLMAN'S	317		11.8	63.3	1.8
with a hint of sage & onion					
flavour, sachet OXO	316		11.1	54.2	6.1
Chicken Stock Cubes					
prepared (100ml) KNORR		7	0.1	0.6	0.4
prepared (100ml) OXO		8	0.4	1.4	0.1
Chilli Paste, Hot					
Very Lazy ENGLISH PROVENDER CO.	67		2	6.7	3.7
Chilli Purée					
GIA	56		3.4	2	19.8
Garlic Paste					
Very Lazy ENGLISH PROVENDER CO.	134		4.9	11.3	7.7
Garlic Purée	423		2.7	13	40
GIA	391		3.3	1.6	41.3
Gravy Instant Granules	462		4.4	40.6	32.5
made up with water	34		0.3	3	2.4
Green Curry Paste					
BLUE DRAGON	96		2.5	8.7	4.5

Food Type	cal per 100g	cal per portion	pro (g)	carb (g)	fat (g)
Ham Stock Cubes					
prepared (100ml) KNORR		7	0.3	0.4	0.4
Lamb Gravy Mix					
with a hint of garden mint,					
sachet OXO	349		9.6	60.3	7.7
and mint, sachet COLMAN'S	316		15.7	59	1.9
Lamb Stock Cubes					
prepared (100ml) KNORR		7	0.2	0.3	0.5
prepared (100ml) OXO		9	0.4	1.7	0.1
Madeira Wine Gravy Mix,					
bonne cuisine					
as prepared CROSSE & BLACKWELL	40		0.9	7.8	0.6
Onion Gravy Granules					
as sold BISTO	391		2.4	62.3	14.7
Passata					
NAPOLINA	25		1.4	4.5	0.1
Organic MERIDIAN FOODS	28		1.2	4.8	0.5
Pork Stock Cubes					
prepared (100ml) KNORR		8	0.3	0.4	0.5
Red Curry Paste					
BLUE DRAGON	97		2.9	9.6	5.2
Roast Beef Flavour Gravy					
Granules					
as sold BISTO	313		2.9	65.6	4.3

Food Type	cal per 100g	cal per portion	pro (g)	carb (g)	fat (g)
Roast Beef Gravy Mix					
as sold SCHWARTZ	306		11.2	58.8	2.9
Roast Chicken Flavour Gravy Granules					
as sold BISTO	310		3.1	64.7	4.4
Roast Chicken Gravy Mix					
as sold SCHWARTZ	189		10.3	23.6	5.9
Roast Lamb Gravy Mix					
as sold SCHWARTZ	336		10.4	63.6	4.5
Roast Onion Flavour Gravy Granules					
as sold BISTO	333		2	66.9	6.4
Roast Onion Gravy Mix					
as sold SCHWARTZ	315		8.8	61	4
Roast Pork Flavour Gravy Granules					
as sold BISTO	314		4.3	64.1	4.5
Roast Pork & Sage Gravy Mix					
as sold SCHWARTZ	354		11.8	63.8	5.8
Roast Turkey Gravy Mix					
as sold SCHWARTZ	337		12.2	56.8	6.8
Roast Vegetables Flavour Gravy Granules					
as sold BISTO	312		3	62.4	5.6

Food Type	cal per 100g	cal per portion	pro (g)	carb (g)	fat (g)
Stock Pot					
beef, as prepared (100ml) KNORR		5	0.1	0.2	0.4
chicken, as prepared (100ml)					
KNORR		5	0.1	0.3	0.4
vegetable, as prepared					
(100ml) KNORR		6	0.1	0.3	0.5
Tomato Purée	76		5	14.2	0.3
HEINZ	57		3.7	10.1	0.2
NAPOLINA	73		4.7	12.6	0.4
Sun-Dried GIA	204		2.6	Tr	21.6
Turkey Gravy Granules					
as sold BISTO	377		2.4	57.2	15.5
Vegetable Granulated Stock					
KNORR	199		8.5	39.9	0.6
Vegetable Gravy Granules					
as sold BISTO	380		2.1	63	13.3
Vegetable Stock					
VECON	125		16.6	13.9	1.3
Vegetable Stock Cubes					
prepared (100ml) KNORR		7	0.1	0.4	0.5
prepared (100ml) OXO		8	0.3	1.5	0.1
Liquid or Concentrated **Bouillons & Gravies**					
Beef Concentrated Liquid Stock					
OXO	148		10.2	26.3	0.3

Food Type	cal per 100g	cal per portion	pro (g)	carb (g)	fat (g)
Beef Gravy					
AINSLEY HARRIOTT	24		0.3	5.3	0.2
Beef Gravy, Rich					
SCHWARTZ	31		0.8	3.4	1.6
Chicken Concentrated Liquid Stock					
OXO	173		6.9	29.1	3.3
Chicken Gravy					
AINSLEY HARRIOTT	23		0.4	5.2	0.1
Chicken Gravy, Rich					
SCHWARTZ	27		0.8	3.3	1.2
Heat & Pour Gravy					
beef BISTO	28		1.8	4.6	0.3
chicken BISTO	35		0.9	3.1	2.1
Lamb Concentrated Liquid Stock					
OXO	194		6.9	37.8	1.6
Lamb Gravy					
AINSLEY HARRIOTT	27		0.5	6	0.1
Onion Concentrated Gravy					
as prepared JUST BOUILLON	52		2	7.8	1.4
Onion Gravy, Rich					
SCHWARTZ	24		0.4	4.3	0.6
Poultry Concentrated Gravy					
as prepared JUST BOUILLON	62		1.8	9.2	2

Food Type	cal per 100g	cal per portion	pro (g)	carb (g)	fat (g)
Red Meat Concentrated Gravy					
as prepared JUST BOUILLON	43		2.6	7.6	0.2
Simply Stock					
beef KNORR	6		1.4	0.1	Tr
chicken KNORR	6		1.6	0.1	Tr
vegetable KNORR	3		0.3	0.5	Tr
Touch of Taste Bouillon					
beef KNORR	73		7.5	9.5	0.5
chicken KNORR	75		4	8	3
vegetable KNORR	101		7.5	17	0.3
Turkey Gravy, Rich					
SCHWARTZ	31		1.9	3.1	1.2
Vegetable Concentrated Liquid Stock					
OXO	216		1.9	45.2	3.1
Stuffings					
Apricot & Orange Stuffing Mix					
PAXO	157		3.8	30.9	2
Breadcrumbs, Golden					
PAXO	354		11.5	73.5	1.6
Breadcrumbs, Natural					
PAXO	353		11.5	73.4	1.4
Chestnut & Cranberry Stuffing Mix					
PAXO	131		3.5	24.1	2.2

Food Type	cal per 100g	cal per portion	pro (g)	carb (g)	fat (g)
Couscous Stuffing Mix					
Crackin' Cranberry, per serving AINSLEY HARRIOTT		56	2.2	10.3	0.7
Fabulously Flavoured Moroccan Magic, per serving AINSLEY HARRIOTT		60	2.7	10.7	0.7
Luscious Lemon, Onion & Thyme, per serving AINSLEY HARRIOTT		60	2.7	10.8	0.7
Scruptious Sage & Onion, per serving AINSLEY HARRIOTT		55	2.6	9.7	0.6
Cranberry, Orange & Chestnut Stuffing Mix					
SHROPSHIRE SPICE CO.	169		6.4	32.5	1.5
Crumb Dressing					
RUSKOLINE	344		11.3	70.6	1.8
Parsley & Thyme Stuffing Mix					
NORFOLK	121		3.3	23.4	1.5
Sage, Red Pepper & Shallot Stuffing Mix					
SHROPSHIRE SPICE CO.	150		6.2	27.9	1.5
Sage & Onion Stuffing Mix					
	269		6.1	29	15.1
NORFOLK	109		3.6	19.8	1.7
PAXO	116		3.2	22.1	1.7

Food Type	cal per 100g	cal per portion	pro (g)	carb (g)	fat (g)
SHROPSHIRE SPICE CO.	155		6.5	29.1	1.4
With Apple PAXO	113		3.1	22.2	1.3
With Garlic PAXO	130		4.1	24.9	1.4
With Lemon PAXO	122		3.4	24.2	1.2
Sausagemeat & Thyme Stuffing Mix					
PAXO	162		7.1	25.3	3.6
Stovetop Chicken Stuffing Mix					
KRAFT	170		4	21	9
Wild Sage & Red Onion Stuffing Mix					
PAXO	148		4.6	28.6	1.7
Dressings					
Balsamic Vinaigrette					
HELLMANN'S	342		0.1	9.6	2.7
Blue Cheese Dressing	345		2.7	19	28.6
Caesar Dressing					
HELLMANN'S	494		2.5	3.5	52.2
WEIGHTWATCHERS	65		3.3	14.7	0.9
Light KRAFT	95		1.7	13	3.6
Warm HELLMANN'S	538		4.5	7.9	54.2
Deli Mayo					
Moroccan style HEINZ	532		0.9	4.6	56.5
roasted garlic HEINZ	537		1.1	5.5	56.6
sun-dried tomato HEINZ	589		1.3	4.9	62.5

Food Type	cal per 100g	cal per portion	pro (g)	carb (g)	fat (g)
tikka style HEINZ	532		0.9	4.6	56.5
French Dressing					
HELLMANN'S	297		0.4	14.9	25.9
WEIGHTWATCHERS	48		0.4	9.7	0.8
Light KRAFT	37		0.1	8.4	Tr
Organic MERIDIAN FOODS	389		0.6	19.7	32.8
Garlic & Herb Dressing					
HELLMANN'S	233		0.7	13.1	19.3
Herb 'n' Garlic Dressing					
light KRAFT	116		1.2	15.5	5.1
Honey & Mustard Dressing					
HELLMANN'S	214		0.9	16.1	15.8
light KRAFT	126		1.2	19	4.6
Italian Dressing					
Classic KRAFT	119		0.1	5.6	10.5
Light KRAFT	29		0.1	6.2	Tr
Warm HELLMANN'S	411		2.1	13.9	38.5
Mayola					
egg- & dairy-free GRANOVITA	449		2	9	45
Mayonnaise	691		1.1	1.7	75.6
HEINZ	663		0.9	3	71.8
HELLMANN'S	707		1.1	1.5	79.1
Dijon mustard HELLMANN'S	194		2.9	3.5	19.6
Dressing WEIGHTWATCHERS	290		1.2	6.9	29.7

Food Type	cal per 100g	cal per portion	pro (g)	carb (g)	fat (g)
Extra Light HELLMANN'S	96		0.6	12	5
Extra Virgin Olive Oil HELLMANN'S	722		1.1	1.5	79.1
Garlic, Organic BAXTERS	759		1.1	4.5	81.8
Lemon, Organic BAXTERS	760		1	14.4	92
Light HEINZ	285		1	9.3	26.8
Light HELLMANN'S	298		0.7	6.5	29.8
Organic BAXTERS	757		1	1.3	81.8
Organic MERIDIAN FOODS	636		0.8	5.7	67.8
Salad Cream	320		2.3	17	27
reduced fat	109		0.8	13	6
HEINZ	332		1.5	20	26.8
WEIGHTWATCHERS	115		1.5	16.2	4.4
Extra Light HEINZ	138		1.9	15.1	7.2
Light HEINZ	244		1.9	13	20
Organic MERIDIAN FOODS	312		1.4	13	28.3
Seafood Sauce					
BAXTERS	528		1.4	9	54
COLMAN'S	296		0.9	21.5	22.9
Thousand Island Dressing					
HELLMANN'S	239		1	13.6	19.6
Classic KRAFT	380		1	20	32.5
Light KRAFT	94		0.6	21.5	0.2
Vinaigrette					
fat-free HELLMANN'S	49		0.1	10.9	0

Food Type	cal per 100g	cal per portion	pro (g)	carb (g)	fat (g)
Chutneys & Pickles					
Albert's Victorian Chutney					
BAXTERS	153		0.9	36.4	0.4
Apple Chutney	190		0.9	49.2	0.2
Apple Cider & Fig Chutney					
BAXTERS	146		0.8	35.2	0.2
Apple & Onion Sweet Chutney					
GARNER'S	179		0.6	44	0.1
Beetroot Pickie					
BRANSTON	123		1.2	28.2	0.3
Branston Pickle					
CROSSE & BLACKWELL	109		0.8	26.1	0.2
small chunk CROSSE & BLACKWELL	109		0.8	26.1	0.2
smooth CROSSE & BLACKWELL	125		0.9	29.8	0.2
Branston Relish					
chilli & jalapeño CROSSE & BLACKWELL	124		1.6	27.8	0.7
gherkin CROSSE & BLACKWELL	149		0.4	36.7	0.1
sweet onion CROSSE & BLACKWELL	153		1	36.3	0.4
tomato & pepper CROSSE & BLACKWELL	159		1.3	37.4	0.4
Brinjal Pickle					
PATAK	367		2.2	34.6	24.4
Cabbage, Pickled					
GARNER'S	65		0.9	14.9	0.2

Food Type	cal per 100g	cal per portion	pro (g)	carb (g)	fat (g)
Capers					
in white wine vinegar OPIES	20		2	1.2	0.8
Chilli Pickle					
PATAK	325		4.3	1.3	33.7
Chilli & Lime Marinated Beetroot					
BAXTERS	106		1.4	9.4	7
Cranberry & Caramelised Red Onion Chutney					
BAXTERS	154		0.3	38	0.1
Crushed Pineapple & Sweet Pepper Chutney					
BAXTERS	163		1.1	28	5.2
Eggs, Pickled					
GARNER'S	83		7.1	0.3	5.9
Fire Roasted Pepper Chutney with Capers					
BAXTERS	170		1	40	0.7
Garlic & Rosemary Marinated Beetroot					
BAXTERS	106		1.5	9.2	7
Gherkins					
pickled	14		0.9	2.6	0.1
Cocktail OPIES	25		0.7	5.6	0.2
Whole HAYWARD'S	34		0.9	5.5	0.5

Food Type

Food Type	cal per 100g	cal per portion	pro (g)	carb (g)	fat (g)
Lime Pickle, Medium Hot					
PATAK	194		2.2	4	18.7
Mango Chutney					
GARNER'S	205		0.8	50	0.2
Bengal Spice SHARWOOD	285		0.3	70.2	0.3
Green Label SHARWOOD	278		0.3	68.5	0.3
Hot PATAK	270		0.3	60.7	0.2
Major Grey PATAK	260		0.4	57.8	0.2
Spiced BAXTERS	173		0.5	42	0.3
Mixed Pickle					
HAYWARD'S	18		1.4	2.4	0.3
Mustard Pickle					
mild HEINZ	123		2.1	24.4	1.2
Onions, pickled					
drained	31		1.5	6	0.1
BARTON'S	19		0.4	4.2	0
GARNER'S	55		0.8	12.8	0.1
HAYWARD'S	23		0.7	4.8	0.1
In balsamic vinegar OPIES	11		1	1.7	0.1
Cocktail OPIES	36		0.6	8.3	Tr
Silverskin GARNER'S	85		0.8	20.3	0.1
Silverskin HAYWARD'S	10		0.4	1.8	0.1
Sweet GARNER'S	97		0.7	23.3	0.1
Sweet HAYWARD'S	21		0.4	4.5	0.1

Food Type	cal per 100g	cal per portion	pro (g)	carb (g)	fat (g)
Piccalilli					
GARNER'S	101		1.4	23	0.4
HAYWARD'S	70		1.4	14.9	0.5
Spreadable BARTON'S	47		0.8	9.6	0.6
Spreadable Sweet HAYWARD'S	105		1.2	24.4	0.3
Traditional BARTON'S	46		0.8	9.4	0.6
Ploughman's Pickle					
HEINZ	117		0.8	26.7	0.2
Red Cabbage					
sliced, pickled HAYWARD'S	14		0.9	2.2	0.2
Sandwich Pickle, tangy					
HEINZ	134		0.7	31.4	0.2
Sauerkraut	9		1.1	1.1	Tr
GUNDELSHEIM	21		1.3	3	0.3
KAUFFMANN	29		1.3	2.3	0.3
Shallots, pickled					
GARNER'S	76		0.9	17.9	0.1
Spanish Tomato & Black Olive Chutney					
BAXTERS	133		1.8	29	1.1
Spiced Fruit Chutney					
BAXTERS	145		0.6	34.9	0.3
Sweet Caramelised Onion Chutney with Orange					
BAXTERS	178		0.6	43	0.4

Food Type

Food Type	cal per 100g	cal per portion	pro (g)	carb (g)	fat (g)
Sweet Cherry Tomato & Peppadew Chutney					
BAXTERS	167		0.8	40.1	0.4
Sweet Pequante Peppers, whole, mild or hot					
PEPPADEW	118		1	28	0.2
Sweet Pickle	109		0.3	27	Tr
Tomato Chutney	128		1.2	31	0.2
BAXTERS	158		1.7	37.1	0.3
Walnuts, pickled, drained					
OPIES	120		0.9	27.5	1.4

Food Type	cal per 100g	cal per portion	pro (g)	carb (g)	fat (g)
Cooking Sauces & Marinades					
Traditional					
Béchamal Sauce					
as prepared CROSSE & BLACKWELL	72		3.7	9.4	2.2
as prepared KNORR	94		1.9	13	3.8
sachet SCHWARTZ	434		11.5	45.6	22.9
Beef Casserole Mix					
sachet COLMAN'S	316		8.6	68.2	1
Beef & Ale Casserole Sauce Mix					
sachet COLMAN'S	320		9.2	66.3	2
Beef & Ale Cook-In-Sauce					
HOMEPRIDE	52		0.7	12	0.1
Beef in Ale Cooking Sauce					
rich BISTO	28		1.8	5	Tr
Bread Sauce					
made with semi-skimmed milk	97		4.2	15.3	2.5
made with whole milk	110		4.1	15.2	4
Bread Sauce Mix					
sachet COLMAN'S	326		8.1	65.1	3.7
Bread Sauce Mix, Luxury					
sachet COLMAN'S	369		12.3	54.8	11.1
sachet SCHWARTZ	355		12.9	61.5	6.4
Cheddar Cheese Sauce Mix					
sachet COLMAN'S	410		19.2	48.5	15.4

Food Type	cal per 100g	cal per portion	pro (g)	carb (g)	fat (g)
sachet SCHWARTZ	361		18.4	55.1	7.4
Cheese & Bacon Pasta Bake					
HOMEPRIDE	67		0.9	3.8	5.3
Cheese & Ham Potato Bake					
HOMEPRIDE	103		1.5	3.8	9.1
Cheese Sauce Granules					
as sold BISTO	483		7	51.9	27.4
Cheese Sauce Packet Mix					
made with semi-skimmed milk	91		5.5	9.2	3.8
made with whole milk	111		5.4	9	6
Chicken Casserole Mix					
sachet SCHWARTZ	344		10.4	63.2	5.6
Chicken Casserole Mix, Traditional					
sachet COLMAN'S	311		5.7	69.4	1.3
Chicken Supreme Casserole Mix					
sachet COLMAN'S	378		12.4	53.9	12.5
Chicken Supreme Cook-In-Sauce					
HOMEPRIDE	126		0.7	4.5	11.5
Chicken & Mushroom Pie Casserole Mix					
sachet COLMAN'S	384		12.4	55.4	12.5
Cottage Pie Sauce Mix					
sachet COLMAN'S	279		13.7	52.5	1.5

Food Type	cal per 100g	cal per portion	pro (g)	carb (g)	fat (g)
Country Vegetable Chicken Cooking Sauce					
BISTO	32		1.2	5.6	0.5
Creamy Cheese & Bacon Pasta Sauce Mix					
sachet COLMAN'S	364		16.7	56.1	8.1
Creamy Cheese & Ham Potato Bake					
HOMEPRIDE	101		1.5	3.6	8.9
Creamy Leek Potato Bake					
HOMEPRIDE	82		1	4.7	6.6.
Creamy Mushroom Chicken Tonight Sauce					
KNORR	81		0.8	5.4	6.3
low-fat KNORR	47		0.7	5.8	2.3
Creamy Mushroom & White Wine Cooking Sauce					
free from MERIDIAN FOODS	117		2.3	5.9	9
Creamy Parsley Sauce Mix					
sachet SCHWARTZ	371		11.5	57.2	10.7
Creamy Pepper Sauce Mix					
sachet SCHWARTZ	342		17.9	52	6.9
Creamy Pepper & Mushroom Sauce Mix					
sachet COLMAN'S	332		9.6	64.6	3.8

Food Type	cal per 100g	cal per portion	pro (g)	carb (g)	fat (g)
Creamy Tomato & Herb Pasta Bake					
HOMEPRIDE	102		1.7	6.5	7.7
Cumberland Sausage & Onion Cooking Sauce					
BISTO	41		1.4	6.8	0.8
Four Cheese Sauce Mix					
sachet COLMAN'S	531		15.1	34.2	37.1
Garlic & Herb Potato Bake					
HOMEPRIDE	104		0.7	5.3	8.9
Hearty Cumberland Sausages Tonight Sauce					
KNORR	35		0.8	7.8	0.1
Hollandaise Sauce for Fish					
as sold SCHWARTZ	152		0.7	0.4	16.4
Hollandaise Sauce Mix					
sachet COLMAN'S	372		6.4	61.6	11.1
Honey & Mustard Chicken Tonight Sauce					
KNORR	104		1.2	12.8	5.3
low-fat KNORR	74		1.1	12.3	2.3
Honey & Mustard Heat & Pour Sauce					
SCHWARTZ	104		0.7	10.1	6.8

Food Type	cal per 100g	cal per portion	pro (g)	carb (g)	fat (g)
Hunter's BBQ Chicken Sauce Mix					
sachet COLMAN'S	344		5.6	77.5	1.3
Lamb Casserole Mix					
sachet SCHWARTZ	297		5.7	61	3.4
Lamb Hotpot Casserole Mix					
sachet COLMAN'S	297		9.7	59.4	2.3
Lamb & Rosemary Casserole Cook-In-Sauce					
HOMEPRIDE	41		0.9	8.9	0.2
Leek & Mustard Sausage Casserole Mix					
sachet SCHWARTZ	275		12.4	50.1	2.7
Lemon Butter Sauce for Fish					
as sold SCHWARTZ	357		6.1	65.3	8
Liver & Bacon Casserole Mix					
sachet COLMAN'S	303		10.3	61.6	1.7
Mushroom Heat & Pour Sauce					
SCHWARTZ	122		1.2	3.9	11.3
Mushroom Sauce Mix, Luxury					
sachet COLMAN'S	481		11.1	35.6	32.7
Onion Sauce					
made with semi-skimmed milk	88		3	8.2	5.1
made with whole milk	101		2.9	8.1	6.6

Food Type	cal per 100g	cal per portion	pro (g)	carb (g)	fat (g)
Onion Sauce Mix					
sachet COLMAN'S	325		9.1	69.4	1.3
Parsley Sauce Granules					
as sold BISTO	487		3.3	54.4	28.5
Parsley Sauce Mix					
sachet COLMAN'S	313		7.2	68	1.4
Peppercorn Chicken Tonight Sauce					
KNORR	91		0.3	4.9	7.8
Peppercorn Pour Over Sauce, Green & Black					
LOYD GROSSMAN	80		1.2	0.5	3.9
Peppercorn Sauce Mix					
sachet COLMAN'S	406		13	49.2	17.5
Pork Casserole Mix					
sachet COLMAN'S	325		5.9	72.3	1.4
Red Wine Cook-In-Sauce					
HOMEPRIDE	48		0.4	9.3	0.5
Red Wine & Onion Sausages Tonight Sauce					
KNORR	35		0.5	7.8	0.2
Rich Sausage & Onion Casserole Sauce Mix					
sachet COLMAN'S	318		9.6	64.2	2.6

Food Type	cal per 100g	cal per portion	pro (g)	carb (g)	fat (g)
Roast Chicken Hearty Casserole Cook-In-Sauce					
HOMEPRIDE	36		0.8	3	0.2
Roasted Garlic & Herb Coating Mix					
BATCHELORS	316		9.5	47.1	11.4
Sausage Casserole Classic Creations Mix					
as sold, CROSSE & BLACKWELL	320		8.3	62.4	4.1
Sausage Casserole Cook-In-Sauce					
HOMEPRIDE	42		0.7	9.4	0.2
Sausage Casserole Mix					
sachet COLMAN'S	324		9.3	68.9	1.2
sachet SCHWARTZ	275		12.4	50.1	2.7
Savoury Mince Casserole Mix					
sachet SCHWARTZ	336		13.1	65.3	2.2
Shepherd's Pie Classic Creations Mix					
as sold CROSSE & BLACKWELL	302		9	53.4	5.8
Shepherd's Pie Cook-In-Sauce					
HOMEPRIDE	41		1.2	8.6	0.2
Shepherd's Pie Sauce Mix					
sachet COLMAN'S	288		11.8	56.7	1.5

Food Type	cal per 100g	cal per portion	pro (g)	carb (g)	fat (g)
Somerset Port Casserole Mix					
sachet SCHWARTZ	320		9.4	61.9	3.8
Somerset Pork Cook-In-Sauce					
HOMEPRIDE	63		0.6	7.1	3.4
Steak & Ale Flavour Pie Sauce Mix, Easy					
sachet COLMAN'S	327		10.2	67.8	1.6
Tomato & Bacon Pasta Bake					
HOMEPRIDE	90		1.5	5.8	6.8
Traditional Chicken Dry Casserole Mix					
sachet COLMAN'S	311		5.7	69.4	1.3
Traditional Sausage Dry Casserole Mix					
sachet COLMAN'S	324		9.3	68.9	1.2
Tuna Pasta Bake Sauce					
HOMEPRIDE	80		1.6	5.6	5.7
Tuna & Pasta Bake Sauce Mix					
sachet COLMAN'S	323		9.2	60	5.2
White Sauce Granules					
as sold BISTO	496		3.2	57.4	28.2
White Sauce Mix, Savoury					
sachet COLMAN'S	428		9.2	57.9	17.7

Food Type	cal per 100g	cal per portion	pro (g)	carb (g)	fat (g)
White Wine & Cream Cook-in-Sauce					
HOMEPRIDE	81		1	8	4.1
Wholegrain Mustard Pour Over Sauce					
LOYD GROSSMAN	83		2	1.3	1.5
Chinese					
Black Bean Stir Fry Sauce					
BLUE DRAGON	95		2.3	18.2	1.1
SHARWOOD	98		2.2	18.8	1.5
Black Bean Stir Fry Sensations, Crushed					
AMOY	100		2.4	16.9	2.9
Black Bean with Roasted Garlic & Chilli Stir Fry Sauce					
BLUE DRAGON	102		2.5	15.6	3.1
Black Bean & Red Pepper Cooking Sauce					
SHARWOOD	62		1.9	10.5	1.4
Cantonese Sauce					
UNCLE BEN'S	86		0.8	20.3	0.2
Chilli & Garlic Sauce					
LEA & PERRINS	60		1	14.9	n/a
Chinese 5 Spice Stir it Up					
KNORR	253		3.2	18.7	18.4

Food Type	cal per 100g	cal per portion	pro (g)	carb (g)	fat (g)
Chinese Szechuan Cooking Sauce					
WEIGHTWATCHERS	48		1.2	7.7	1.4
Chow Mein Mix					
ROSS	58		2.2	13.3	0.4
Chow Mein Stir Fry Sauce					
BLUE DRAGON	91		1.1	14.1	3.2
Golden Plum, Ginger & Chilli Sauce					
BLUE DRAGON	178		0.5	43	0
Hoi Sin Sauce					
BLUE DRAGON	276		0.4	63.1	2.5
SHARWOOD	149		1.5	33.3	0.5
Hoi Sin Sauce for Spare Ribs					
SHARWOOD	149		1.5	33.3	0.5
Hoi Sin & Garlic Stir Fry Sauce					
BLUE DRAGON	146		1.5	27.8	3
Hoi Sin & Plum Cooking Sauce					
SHARWOOD	94		0.7	19.9	1.3
Hoi Sin & Sesame Sauce					
BLUE DRAGON	187		3.5	39	1.9
Hoi Sin & Spring Onion Stir Fry Sauce					
SHARWOOD	119		1.3	26.5	0.9

Food Type	cal per 100g	cal per portion	pro (g)	carb (g)	fat (g)
Honey & Cashew Sauce					
BLUE DRAGON	129		1.8	28.3	1
Hong Kong Curry Oriental Sauce					
LOYD GROSSMAN	106		1.3	7.8	7.7
Kung Po Cooking Sauce					
SHARWOOD	175		0.6	41.2	0.9
Lemon Chicken Sauce					
UNCLE BEN'S	95		0.3	22.6	0.3
Lemon & Sesame Stir Fry Sauce					
SHARWOOD	125		0.1	30.9	0.1
Light Soy Sauce					
SHARWOOD	37		2.7	6.4	0.2
Oriental Beef Stir Fry Creations					
as sold CROSSE & BLACKWELL	350		9	66	5.3
Oriental Chicken Stir Fry Creations					
as sold CROSSE & BLACKWELL	335		6.1	70.9	2.8
Oriental Sweet & Sour Cooking Sauce					
WEIGHTWATCHERS	51		0.8	11.7	0.1
Oyster Sauce					
BLUE DRAGON	121		3.4	26.9	Tr
SHARWOOD	98		0.9	23	0.2

Food Type	cal per 100g	cal per portion	pro (g)	carb (g)	fat (g)
Oyster & Spring Onion Stir Fry Sauce					
BLUE DRAGON	108		1.1	25.1	0.1
Pad Thai Sauce					
BLUE DRAGON	222		2	40	6
Peking Lemon Stir Fry Sauce					
BLUE DRAGON	133		Tr	31.2	0.8
Plum Sauce					
BLUE DRAGON	243		0.2	60.3	0.1
SHARWOOD	240		0.2	59.5	0.1
Rich Hoi Sin & Red Onion Stir Fry Sensations					
AMOY	130		2.6	23.9	2.5
Rich Mushroom & Oyster Stir Fry Sensations					
AMOY	106		3.1	21.9	0.5
Soy, Sesame & Ginger Sauce for Fish					
as sold SCHWARTZ	93		1.3	18.8	1.4
Spare Rib Sauce					
BLUE DRAGON	198		1.4	47.1	0.4
Spicy Szechuan Tomato Stir Fry Sauce					
BLUE DRAGON	121		1.4	16.2	5.4

Food Type	cal per 100g	cal per portion	pro (g)	carb (g)	fat (g)
Spicy Tomato Szechuan Stir Fry Sauce					
SHARWOOD	79		1.3	17.5	0.3
Spring Roll Sauce					
BLUE DRAGON	220		0.3	54.7	Tr
Sticky Plum Stir Fry Sauce					
BLUE DRAGON	242		0.1	35.6	0.3
Succulent Szechuan Tomato Stir Fry Sensations					
AMOY	111		1.4	23.1	1
Sweet & Sour Chicken Tonight Sauce					
KNORR	75		0.6	17.8	0.1
Sweet & Sour Cook-In Sauce					
HOMEPRIDE	95		0.3	23.1	0.1
Sweet & Sour Cooking Sauce					
SHARWOOD	105		0.6	24.5	0.5
Sweet & Sour Sauce					
BLUE DRAGON	201		0.7	49.4	0.1
UNCLE BEN'S	88		0.4	20.9	0.2
Extra Spicy UNCLE BEN'S	89		0.4	20.9	0.2
Light UNCLE BEN'S	52		0.4	11.6	0.1
Organic SEEDS OF CHANGE	100		0.4	24.4	0.1
With Extra Pineapple UNCLE BEN'S	89		0.3	21.2	0.2

Food Type	cal per 100g	cal per portion	pro (g)	carb (g)	fat (g)
Sweet & Sour Sauce Mix					
sachet COLMAN'S	328		2.3	78.6	0.5
Sweet & Sour Sizzle & Stir					
KNORR	151		0.5	16.7	9.1
Sweet & Sour Stir Fry Sauce					
BLUE DRAGON	127		0.5	22	3.6
SHARWOOD	112		0.5	27.2	0.1
Sweet & Sour Stir Fry Sauce, Aromatic					
AMOY	195		0.4	46.8	0.3
Sweet Chilli Sauce					
BLUE DRAGON	206		0.8	49.4	0.6
SHARWOOD	182		0.7	43.7	0.3
Sweet Chilli & Garlic Stir Fry Sauce					
BLUE DRAGON	160		0.2	38.1	0.6
Sweet Chilli & Red Pepper Cooking Sauce					
SHARWOOD	70		0.6	16.6	0.1
Sweet Soy & Spring Onion Stir Fry Sensations					
AMOY	195		2	31.5	6.5
Szechuan Chilli Sauce					
UNCLE BEN'S	90		1	11.3	4.5

Food Type	cal per 100g	cal per portion	pro (g)	carb (g)	fat (g)
Teriyaki Marinade					
BLUE DRAGON	263		3.4	62.3	Tr
Teriyaki Stir Fry Sauce					
BLUE DRAGON	109		0.4	26.4	Tr
Teriyaki with Black Pepper Stir Fry Sauce					
SHARWOOD	96		0.9	22.5	0.3
Yellow Bean Stir Fry Sauce					
SHARWOOD	104		1.1	23.5	0.6
Zesty Lemon & Black Pepper Stir Fry Sensations					
AMOY	102		0.2	24.4	0.1
Italian					
Amatriciana	155		4.4	5	13
Arrabbiata, fresh	48		1.2	7	1.7
Basil & Oregano Sauce					
RAGU	36		1.2	7.5	0.1
Bolognese Sauce					
fresh, with beef	77		4.7	3.4	5
DOLMIO	52		1.7	8.7	1.2
LOYD GROSSMAN	75		2	10.2	2.9
RAGU	33		0.2	7	0.1
Express Sauce DOLMIO	88		7.4	7.1	3.3

Food Type	cal per 100g	cal per portion	pro (g)	carb (g)	fat (g)
Express Sauce Extra Onion & Garlic DOLMIO	89		7.4	7.3	3.3
Express Sauce with Extra Mushroom DOLMIO	91		7.8	7.4	3.3
Extra Chunky Mediterranean Vegetables DOLMIO	51		1.6	7.9	1.4
Extra Chunky Sweet Pepper DOLMIO	52		1.5	8.5	1.3
Extra Mushroom DOLMIO	48		1.5	7.6	1.3
Extra Onion & Garlic DOLMIO	50		1.5	8.1	1.3
Extra Spicy DOLMIO	48		1.5	7.7	1.2
Extra Summer Garden Vegetables DOLMIO	40		1.4	6	0.3
Extra Winter Vegetables DOLMIO	49		1.5	7.7	1.3
Original, Light DOLMIO	33		1.5	5.7	0.2
Spicy RAGU	36		1.2	7.6	0.1
Traditional, Organic SEEDS OF CHANGE	58		1.3	10.4	1.2
Carbonara					
fresh	196		6	4.8	17
fresh, low fat	81		5	5	4.5
Carbonara Pasta Bake					
HOMEPRIDE	111		0.8	3.5	10.4

Food Type	cal per 100g	cal per portion	pro (g)	carb (g)	fat (g)
Carbonara Pasta Sauce					
LOYD GROSSMAN	123		2.8	7.5	9.1
NAPOLINA	150		3.9	4.8	12.8
Chargrilled Vegetable Sauce					
BERTOLLI	48		1.4	6.2	2
Cherry Tomato & Pesto Stir-in Sauce					
DOLMIO	107		2.1	8.8	7.1
Chunky Vegetable Pasta Sauce					
organic MERIDIAN FOODS	67		1.4	4.1	5
Creamy Carbonara Express Pasta Sauce					
DOLMIO	149		3.4	4.2	13.2
Creamy Carbonara Pasta Bake					
DOLMIO	125		1.4	4.9	11
Creamy Carbonara Stir-in Sauce					
DOLMIO	170		5.6	4.5	14.5
Creamy Mushroom Express Pasta Sauce					
DOLMIO	107		1.4	3.8	9.6
Creamy Sun-Dried Tomato Cooking Sauce					
free from MERIDIAN FOODS	180		1.4	6.7	16.4
Creamy Tomato Pasta Bake					
DOLMIO	102		1.5	8.7	6.8

Cooking Sauces & Marinades

Food Type	cal per 100g	cal per portion	pro (g)	carb (g)	fat (g)
Creamy Tomato & Herb Cooking Sauce					
free from MERIDIAN FOODS	47		1.8	6.1	1.7
Frito, tomato					
HEINZ	73		1.3	7.7	4.1
Lasagne Recipe Mix					
sachet, as sold SCHWARTZ	313		6.6	70.1	0.7
Marinara Pasta Sauce					
BUITONI	64		1	9.6	2.4
Mediterranean Tomato Spread & Bake					
HEINZ	80		1.3	13	2.5
Mediterranean Vegetable Pasta Bake with Crunch Topping					
HOMEPRIDE	63		1.7	13.6	0.2
Mediterranean Vegetable Sauce					
BERTOLLI	88		1.7	4.1	7.2
Mushroom, Garlic, Oregano & Tomato Sauce					
BERTOLLI	90		1.9	3.8	7.5
Onion & Garlic Sauce					
RAGU	34		1.3	7.1	0.1
Pasta 'n' Sauce					
cheese, leek & ham BATCHELORS	379		14.1	68.3	5.5
chicken & mushroom BATCHELORS	361		12.4	73.5	2

Food Type	cal per 100g	cal per portion	pro (g)	carb (g)	fat (g)
macaroni cheese BATCHELORS	372		17.2	65.2	4.7
mild cheese & broccoli BATCHELORS	363		15	67	3.9
mushroom & wine BATCHELORS	369		14.2	68.6	4.2
tomato, onion & herbs BATCHELORS	348		13.8	68.8	2
Pesto					
creamy fresh	45		2.2	6	1.3
jar	374		5	0.8	39
red, jar	358		4.1	3.1	36.6
Green LOYD GROSSMAN	458		4.3	11.9	43.7
Green, Classic SEEDS OF CHANGE	527		4.7	7.5	53.1
Green, Free From MERIDIAN FOODS	519		5.9	5.2	52.6
Red LOYD GROSSMAN	529		5.4	10	51.9
Red, Free From MERIDIAN FOODS	351		3.4	6	35
Rosso BERTOLLI	389		6.6	8.1	36.7
Verdi BERTOLLI	575		5.7	4.3	59.5
Primavera Pasta Sauce					
LOYD GROSSMAN	98		1.4	6.3	7.4
Puttanesca Pasta Sauce					
LOYD GROSSMAN	90		1.7	6.8	6.2
Red Lasagne Sauce					
DOLMIO	55		1.3	9.3	1.3
HOMEPRIDE	44		1.1	9.7	0.1
RAGU	43		1.1	9.7	Tr
Red Wine & Herbs Pasta Sauce					
RAGU	35		1.2	7.4	0.1

Cooking Sauces & Marinades

Food Type	cal per 100g	cal per portion	pro (g)	carb (g)	fat (g)
Rich Tomato with Basil Pesto Express Pasta Sauce					
DOLMIO	86		2	6.2	5.9
Roasted Mediterranean Vegetable Pasta Bake					
DOLMIO	55		2.2	8.8	1.2
Roasted Red Pepper Stir & Serve					
organic SEEDS OF CHANGE	140		1.1	7.5	11.8
Roasted Vegetables Stir-in Sauce					
DOLMIO	133		1.6	8.4	10.3
Sauces in a Pouch					
BERTOLLI	40		2	7	0.5
basil BERTOLLI	44		2	77	0.5
creamy BERTOLLI	62		1.3	7.6	2.9
garlic BERTOLLI	56		1.9	10.5	0.7
spicy BERTOLLI	45		2	7.7	0.6
Signature Fresh Cherry Tomatoes with Basil & Parmesan					
organic SEEDS OF CHANGE	81		2.1	8	4.5
Signature Fresh Cherry Tomatoes & Olive					
organic SEEDS OF CHANGE	72		1.5	8	3.8

Food Type	cal per 100g	cal per portion	pro (g)	carb (g)	fat (g)
Signature Mediterranean Vegetable					
organic SEEDS OF CHANGE	70		1.5	8.3	3.5
Signature Slow Roasted Garlic & Chilli					
organic SEEDS OF CHANGE	73		1.3	8	4.5
Signature Tomato & Roasted Pepper					
organic SEEDS OF CHANGE	85		1.4	8.5	5
Slow Roasted Garlic & Tomato Stir In Sauce					
DOLMIO	134		1.7	9.5	9.9
Smokey Bacon & Tomato Stir In Sauce					
DOLMIO	165		5.5	6.9	12.8
Smokey Bacon Pasta Sauce					
LOYD GROSSMAN	98		3.1	5.4	7.2
Spaghetti Bolognese Sauce Mix					
sachet COLMAN'S	289		10.9	58.2	1.4
Spicy Italian Chilli Express Pasta Sauce					
DOLMIO	51		1.5	7.5	1.6
Spicy Pepperoni & Tomato Stir In Sauce					
DOLMIO	154		3.2	9.3	11.6

Food Type	cal per 100g	cal per portion	pro (g)	carb (g)	fat (g)
Spicy Tomato & Pepperoni Pasta Bake Sauce					
HOMEPRIDE	74		1.8	7.5	4.1
Spicy Tomato & Sweet Onion Stir-in Sauce					
DOLMIO	110		1.6	10.4	6.8
Sun-Dried Tomato Pasta Sauce					
organic MERIDIAN FOODS	61		1.3	3.9	4.5
Sun-Dried Tomato Stir-in Sauce					
DOLMIO	153		1.7	11.1	11.3
light DOLMIO	92		1.7	10.7	4.7
Sun-Dried Tomato & Basil Stir & Serve					
organic SEEDS OF CHANGE	168		1.6	9	14
Sun-Ripened Tomato & Basil Express Pasta Sauce					
DOLMIO	52		1.5	7.9	1.6
Sweet Chilli, Red Onion & Tomato Sauce					
BERTOLLI	91		1.7	4.9	7.2
Sweet Pepper Stir-in Sauce					
DOLMIO	137		1.5	9.7	10.3
Sweet Pepper & Tomato Sauce					
BERTOLLI	89		1.5	4.3	7.2

Food Type	cal per 100g	cal per portion	pro (g)	carb (g)	fat (g)
Sweet Red Pepper Pasta Sauce					
LOYD GROSSMAN	87		1.7	7.3	5.6
Taste of Italy					
Calabria DOLMIO	101		2.8	7.1	6.8
Rome DOLMIO	97		2.1	7.2	6.6
Sicily DOLMIO	67		1.8	7.8	3.2
Sorrento DOLMIO	93		2.8	6.7	6.1
Tuscany DOLMIO	67		1.4	7.4	3
Tomato Pasta Sauce					
jar	47		2	6.9	1.5
Tomato, Garlic & Onion Pasta Sauce					
BUITONI	64		2.4	10	1.6
Tomato, Red Wine & Shallots Pasta Sauce					
BERTOLLI	45		1.5	6	1.7
Tomato, Roasted Garlic & Mushroom Pasta Sauce					
BERTOLLI	45		1.5	5	2.1
Tomato, Romano & Garlic Pasta Sauce					
BERTOLLI	61		2.3	6.4	2.8
Tomato & Basil Sauce					
fresh	51		1.8	8.8	0.9
BERTOLLI	43		1.2	7.3	1

Food Type	cal per 100g	cal per portion	pro (g)	carb (g)	fat (g)
LOYD GROSSMAN	90		1.7	7.9	5.7
Organic MERIDIAN FOODS	58		1.4	4	4.1
Organic SEEDS OF CHANGE	59		1.2	9	2
Tomato & Chargrilled Vegetables Pasta Sauce					
LOYD GROSSMAN	89		1.8	7.9	5.6
Tomato & Cheese Pasta Bake					
DOLMIO	55		2.2	8.8	1.2
Tomato & Chill Pasta Sauce					
LOYD GROSSMAN	88		1.7	7.3	5.7
NAPOLINA	90		1.7	9.2	4.9
Organic MERIDIAN FOODS	58		1.4	4	4.1
Tomato & Herb Pasta Bake					
HOMEPRIDE	102		1.7	6.5	7.7
Tomato & Herb Pasta Sauce					
organic MERIDIAN FOODS	64		1.6	8.1	2.8
Tomato & Mascarpone Sauce					
NAPOLINA	130		2.2	6.5	10.6
Tomato & Mild Chilli Pasta Bake with crunch topping					
HOMEPRIDE	69		1.8	13.9	0.6
Tomato & Mushroom Pasta Sauce					
organic MERIDIAN FOODS	65		1.8	8	2.8

Food Type	cal per 100g	cal per portion	pro (g)	carb (g)	fat (g)
Tomato & Olive Pasta Sauce					
organic MERIDIAN FOODS	64		1.5	7.3	3.2
Tomato & Pepper Pasta Sauce					
organic MERIDIAN FOODS	99		1.5	10.6	5.5
Tomato & Roasted Garlic Pasta Sauce					
LOYD GROSSMAN	92		2	8.8	5.5
Tomato & Wild Mushroom Pasta Sauce					
LOYD GROSSMAN	88		2.1	7.4	5.6
Traditional Pasta Sauce					
RAGU	45		1.6	5.8	1.8
White Lasagne Sauce					
DOLMIO	98		0.5	6.9	7.5
HOMEPRIDE	78		1.2	6.5	5.3
RAGU	158		0.6	4.8	15.2
Indian					
Balti Cooking Sauce					
LOYD GROSSMAN	163		1.7	8.8	13.4
PATAK	70		1.2	5.9	1
SHARWOOD	75		1.6	9.4	3.5
UNCLE BEN'S	75		1.3	7.9	4.2
Organic SEEDS OF CHANGE	72		1.1	7.9	3.9

Food Type	cal per 100g	cal per portion	pro (g)	carb (g)	fat (g)
Bhuna Cooking Sauce					
LOYD GROSSMAN	144		2.6	11.6	9.7
SHARWOOD	79		1	10.9	3.5
Chicken Curry Sauce Mix					
sachet COLMAN'S	374		4.2	63.7	11.4
Chip Shop Curry Granules					
as sold BISTO	427		3.4	63.5	17.7
Chip Shop Curry Sauce Mix					
sachet COLMAN'S	342		3.6	78.8	1.4
Creamy Chicken Curry Sauce Mix					
sachet COLMAN'S	392		10.8	51.2	16
Creamy Curry Chicken Tonight Sauce					
KNORR	78		0.6	2.3	7.4
Curry Cook-In-Sauce					
HOMEPRIDE	68		0.8	10.5	2.5
Curry Paste					
Balti PATAK	388		4	14.6	34
Bhuna PATAK	400		4.3	17.5	34.4
Biryani PATAK	345		5	6	33
Garam Masala PATAK	388		3.4	14.9	34.7
Korma PATAK	303		3.2	11.6	26.3
Madras, Hot PATAK	520		4.8	9.4	51.1
Rogan Josh PATAK	390		4.2	8.9	37.3

Food Type	cal per 100g	cal per portion	pro (g)	carb (g)	fat (g)
Tandoori PATAK	133		3.4	23.1	2
Tikka PATAK	148		3.6	16.9	6.5
Vindaloo PATAK	500		4.9	10	48.7
Curry Sauce					
Canned	78		1.5	7.1	5
Medium UNCLE BEN'S	84		0.9	9.9	4.5
Curry Sauce Mix					
sachet COLMAN'S	353		4.9	80.5	1.2
Dhansak Cooking Sauce					
LOYD GROSSMAN	82		3.4	11.1	2.7
Dhansak Spice & Stir Sauce					
GEETA'S	112		5.1	13.7	5
Dopiaza Cooking Sauce					
LOYD GROSSMAN	92		2.4	12.9	3.4
PATAK	81		1.7	7.5	4.8
Goan Curry Sauce					
GEETA'S	151		1.6	6.2	13.2
Jalfrezi Cooking Sauce					
LOYD GROSSMAN	127		2.1	8.2	9.5
PATAK	112		1.7	9.7	7.2
UNCLE BEN'S	78		1.2	8.6	4.3
Organic SEEDS OF CHANGE	105		1.1	9	7.2
Spicy SHARWOOD	87		1.8	9.2	4.8
Karai Bhuna Spice & Stir Sauce					
GEETA'S	97		1.9	7.2	7

Food Type	cal per 100g	cal per portion	pro (g)	carb (g)	fat (g)
Karai Cooking Sauce					
PATAK	122		3.2	13.7	5.8
Kashmiri Curry Creation Paste					
GEETA'S	92		2	6.6	6.4
Korma Cook-in-Sauce					
HOMEPRIDE	150		1.9	11.6	10.7
Korma Cooking Sauce					
LOYD GROSSMAN	244		3.6	19.1	17
PATAK	176		1.3	9.3	14.8
SHARWOOD	162		1.7	15.9	10.2
UNCLE BEN'S	139		1.3	12	9.5
Free From MERIDIAN FOODS	136		2.4	9	9.9
Lighter SHARWOOD	100		1.5	9.4	6.3
Organic SEEDS OF CHANGE	164		0.7	11	13.1
With Flaked Almonds					
WEIGHTWATCHERS	61		2	8.5	2.1
Korma Sizzle & Stir					
KNORR	253		1.5	11	22.5
Madras Cooking Sauce					
LOYD GROSSMAN	180		2.5	6.8	15.9
PATAK	94		1.9	7.2	6.3
Hot & Spicy, Organic SEEDS					
OF CHANGE	83		1	8.4	5
Madras Spice & Stir Sauce					
GEETA'S	104		1.6	6.1	8.2

Food Type	cal per 100g	cal per portion	pro (g)	carb (g)	fat (g)
Pasanda Cooking Sauce					
PATAK	124		2.3	8.9	8.7
Pudina Tikka Spice & Stir Sauce					
GEETA'S	89		2.2	6.3	6.4
Rogan Josh Cooking Sauce					
LOYD GROSSMAN	194		2.4	10.5	15.8
PATAK	62		1.5	7.8	2.6
SHARWOOD	79		1.6	8	4.5
Saag Spice & Stir Sauce					
GEETA'S	142		3.6	10.5	9.8
Tandoori Marinade Curry Creations Paste					
GEETA'S	157		3	7.6	12.8
Tikka Masala Cooking Sauce					
LOYD GROSSMAN	206		2.6	12.5	16.2
PATAK	96		1.7	6.1	7.2
SHARWOOD	123		1.5	10.8	8.2
UNCLE BEN'S	85		1.5	9.3	4.7
Free From MERIDIAN FOODS	129		1.8	10.7	8.7
Lighter SHARWOOD	75		1.5	7.4	4.4
Organic SEEDS OF CHANGE	115		1.4	8.7	8.3
Spicy SHARWOOD	111		1.7	10.7	6.8
Tikka Masala Sizzle & Stir					
KNORR	201		1.5	11.5	16.6

Food Type	cal per 100g	cal per portion	pro (g)	carb (g)	fat (g)
Tikka Spread & Bake					
HEINZ	87		2.4	10	4.2
Vindaloo Cooking Sauce					
PATAK	119		1.7	8.5	8.6
Mexican & US					
Barbecue Cook-In-Sauce					
HOMEPRIDE	76		0.7	15	1.5
Barbecue Heat & Pour Sauce					
SCHWARTZ	70		0.6	13.4	1.6
BBQ Sprinkle or Marinade Mix					
as sold SCHWARTZ	254		11.8	39.8	5.3
Burrito Spice Mix					
OLD EL PASO	304		13	54	4
Cajun Sauce					
UNCLE BEN'S	57		0.9	8.2	2.3
Cajun Season & Sauce Mix					
DISCOVERY FOODS	68		1.7	11.2	1.8
Cajun Sprinkle or Marinade Mix					
as sold SCHWARTZ	222		12.7	26.2	7.4
Chicken Fajita Casserole Mix					
sachet SCHWARTZ	283		10.9	54.1	2.5
Chicken Fajita Seasoning Mix					
sachet COLMAN'S	344		9.4	62.5	6.3
Chilli Con Carne Casserole Mix					
sachet COLMAN'S	316		10.4	62.9	2.5

Food Type	cal per 100g	cal per portion	pro (g)	carb (g)	fat (g)
sachet SCHWARTZ	293		7.9	57.2	3.6
Chilli Con Carne Casserole Mix, Hot					
sachet SCHWARTZ	258		10.9	43.6	4.5
Chilli Con Carne Sauce					
hot UNCLE BEN'S	59		2.2	11	0.6
medium UNCLE BEN'S	59		2.2	11.2	0.5
mild UNCLE BEN'S	53		1.9	10.3	0.4
Chilli Con Carne Sizzle & Stir					
KNORR	133		4	12.3	7.5
Chilli Cook-In-Sauce					
HOMEPRIDE	65		2.4	10.5	0.6
Chilli Season & Sauce Mix, Hot					
DISCOVERY FOODS	75		3.9	19.6	0.4
Chilli Spice Mix					
OLD EL PASO	299		7	57	5
Chilli with Jalapeño Peppers					
organic SEEDS OF CHANGE	72		2.4	12.5	1.4
Creole Season & Sauce Mix					
DISCOVERY FOODS	66		1.5	10.7	1.7
Enchilada Cooking Sauce					
OLD EL PASO	73		1.6	6	4.8
Enchilada Season & Sauce Mix					
DISCOVERY FOODS	52		1.4	4.8	3

Food Type

Food Type	cal per 100g	cal per portion	pro (g)	carb (g)	fat (g)
Fajita Cooking Sauce					
OLD EL PASO	40		1.6	8.4	0.5
Fajita Season & Sauce Mix					
DISCOVERY FOODS	58		1.9	8.7	1.7
Fajita Spice Mix					
DISCOVERY FOODS	270		9	53	7
OLD EL PASO	306		9	54	6
Mexican Chili Chicken Casserole Mix					
sachet SCHWARTZ	299		7	55.1	5.6
Mexican Fajita Stir it Up					
KNORR	652		5	19.7	61.2
Nachos Kit, Complete					
DISCOVERY FOODS	250		8.5	N/a	6
OLD EL PASO	506		7	61	26
Ranch Barbecue Sausages Tonight Sauce					
KNORR	90		1.8	14.8	2.6
Sticky BBQ Spread & Bake					
HEINZ	168		1	39.6	0.6
Sticky Ribs Sauce					
DISCOVERY FOODS	202		1.1	39.9	4.7
Taco Spice Mix					
DISCOVERY FOODS	240		9.8	31.4	8.4
OLD EL PASO	298		4.6	60	2.6

Food Type	cal per 100g	cal per portion	pro (g)	carb (g)	fat (g)
Texan Barbeque Stir it Up					
KNORR	626		4.3	29.9	54.4
Texas BBQ with Sweet Peppers Sauce					
UNCLE BEN'S	77		1.1	16.4	0.7
European					
Beef Bourguignon Casserole Mix					
sachet COLMAN'S	310		5.4	69.5	1.2
Beef Bourguignon Cook-In-Sauce					
HOMEPRIDE	35		0.5	6.2	0.1
Beef Stroganoff Casserole Mix					
sachet COLMAN'S	355		11.8	49.6	12.2
Bourguignon Beef Tonight					
KNORR	57		0.6	7.6	2.6
Burgundy Red Wine Sauce					
LOYD GROSSMAN	38		0.9	3.4	Tr
Chasseur Cook-In-Sauce					
HOMEPRIDE	43		0.7	9	0.1
Chicken Chasseur Casserole Mix					
sachet COLMAN'S	289		9.4	58.5	2
Chicken Provençal Cook-In-Sauce					
HOMEPRIDE	39		1.1	7.9	0.3

Food Type	cal per 100g	cal per portion	pro (g)	carb (g)	fat (g)
Classic Chasseur Chicken Tonight Sauce					
KNORR	49		0.6	5.3	2.8
Coq au Vin Casserole Mix					
sachet COLMAN'S	311		6.6	66.7	2
sachet SCHWARTZ	321		7.4	68.7	1.8
Country French Chicken Tonight Sauce					
KNORR	84		0.4	4.8	7
low-fat KNORR	45		0.4	4.4	2.9
French White Wine & Tarragon Sauce for Fish					
as sold SCHWARTZ	124		1.1	5	11.1
Mediterranean Sprinkle or Marinade Mix					
as sold SCHWARTZ	273		12.5	38.6	1.9
Moussaka Casserole Mix					
sachet SCHWARTZ	288		8.8	58.6	2
Spanish Chicken, Chicken Tonight Sauce					
KNORR	42		1	6.7	1.3
with red & green peppers KNORR	49		1.2	8	1.3
Stroganoff Cook-In-Sauce					
HOMEPRIDE	83		0.7	5.5	6.3

Food Type	cal per 100g	cal per portion	pro (g)	carb (g)	fat (g)
Swedish Style Meatballs Sauce Mix					
sachet COLMAN'S	407		11	55.7	15.5
World					
Fragrant Thai Green Curry Stir Fry Sensations					
AMOY	83		1.4	17.2	6.9
Green Thai Cooking Sauce					
free from MERIDIAN FOODS	105		1.2	5.7	8.5
Green Thai Curry Sauce					
LOYD GROSSMAN	130		2.3	10.1	9
Indonesian Satay Cooking Sauce					
SHARWOOD	159		5.4	10	10.8
Jamaican Jerk Stir it Up					
KNORR	633		3.9	20.9	59.3
Kaffir Lime & Coriander Stir Fry Sauce					
SHARWOOD	59		0	14.3	0.2
Malaysian Rendang					
LOYD GROSSMAN	168		3.1	10.7	12.5
Oyster & Thai Basil Stir Fry Sauce					
SHARWOOD	63		0	15.2	0.2

Food Type	cal per 100g	cal per portion	pro (g)	carb (g)	fat (g)
Peri-Peri Marinade					
hot NANDO'S	89		Tr	10.9	4.8
lime & coriander NANDO'S	120		Tr	11.9	7.8
sweet & sticky NANDO'S	136		Tr	32.1	0.6
Red Thai Curry Sauce					
LOYD GROSSMAN	123		2.6	11.7	7.3
Roasted Peanut Satay Stir Fry Sensations					
AMOY	221		4.7	21.9	12.4
Royal Thai Green Curry Sauce					
BLUE DRAGON	160		2.3	6.9	13.7
Royal Thai Red Curry Sauce					
BLUE DRAGON	166		1.5	8.8	13.9
Satay Stir Fry Sauce					
BLUE DRAGON	184		4.6	22	8.6
Sweet Chilli & Lemongrass Stir Fry Sauce					
SHARWOOD	82		0.3	19.7	0.1
Sweet Thai Chilli Stir Fry Sensations					
AMOY	147		1	30.9	1.9
Teriyaki Soya Sauce, Natural					
organic MERIDIAN FOODS	101		5	15.3	0.3
Teriyaki Stir Fry Sauce					
BLUE DRAGON	109		0.4	26.4	Tr

Food Type	cal per 100g	cal per portion	pro (g)	carb (g)	fat (g)
Teriyaki with Black Pepper Stir Fry Sauce					
SHARWOOD	96		0.9	22.5	0.3
Teriyaki & Sesame Seeds Stir Fry Sensations					
AMOY	146		1.6	24.6	4.3
Thai Coconut Curry Sauce					
UNCLE BEN'S	108		1.4	13.3	5.3
Thai Green Curry Cooking Sauce					
SHARWOOD	123		1.2	4	11.3
Thai Green Curry Paste					
AMOY	155		1.8	9.1	12.3
SHARWOOD	77		2.5	15.4	0.7
Thai Green Curry Sauce Sizzle & Stir					
KNORR	212		0.8	6.6	20.3
Thai Mussaman Curry Cooking Sauce					
SHARWOOD	98		2.7	10.1	5.3
Thai Red Curry Paste					
AMOY	259		2.1	9.1	23.8
SHARWOOD	117		4	22.1	1.4
Thai Red Curry Sauce					
SHARWOOD	93		1.2	8.1	6.2

Food Type	cal per 100g	cal per portion	pro (g)	carb (g)	fat (g)
Thai Sweet Chilli Sauce					
UNCLE BEN'S	103		0.8	23.6	0.3
Thai Yellow Curry Coookling Sauce					
SHARWOOD	86		1.2	8.8	5.2
Yellow Thai Curry Sauce					
LOYD GROSSMAN	117		1.3	7	9.1

Food Type	cal per 100g	cal per portion	pro (g)	carb (g)	fat (g)
Crisps & Nibbles					
Crisps					
Barbecue Rib Flavour Crisps					
per pack (25g) WALKERS		131	1.6	12.5	8.3
Cheese & Onion Crisps					
per pack (34.5g)					
GOLDENWONDER		178	2	18.1	10.9
per pack (34.5g) WALKERS		181	2.4	17.3	11.4
Baked, per pack (25g) WALKERS		99	1.6	18.3	2.1
Lights, per pack (24g) WALKERS		113	1.8	14.9	5
French Fries					
cheese & onion, per pack (19g)					
WALKERS		82	1	12.5	3
ready salted, per pack (19g)					
WALKERS		81	1	12.4	3
salt & vinegar, per pack (19g)					
WALKERS		82	1	12.5	3
Hula Hoops					
per pack (25g) UNITED BISCUITS		129	1.1	20.5	9.7
BBQ beef, per pack (25g)					
UNITED BISCUITS		128	0.9	15.1	7.1
cheese & onion, per pack (25g)					
UNITED BISCUITS		129	0.9	15.3	7.1
roast chicken, per pack (25g)					
UNITED BISCUITS		129	1	15.2	7.2

Food Type	cal per 100g	cal per portion	pro (g)	carb (g)	fat (g)
salt & vinegar, per pack (25g)					
UNITED BISCUITS		129	0.8	15.5	7.1
smokey bacon, per pack (25g)					
UNITED BISCUITS		128	0.9	15.1	7.1
Kettle Chips					
honey barbecue KETTLE FOODS	465		6.7	53.6	25.2
lightly salted KETTLE FOODS	485		6.3	55.1	26.6
mature cheddar & red onion					
KETTLE FOODS	467		7.5	52.2	25.4
no added salt KETTLE FOODS	486		5.9	56.3	26.3
red Thai curry KETTLE FOODS	467		6.5	52.5	25.8
sea salt & balsamic vinegar					
KETTLE FOODS	489		6.8	53.5	27.5
sea salt with crushed black					
peppercorns KETTLE FOODS	482		6.5	53.8	26.7
sour cream & chive KETTLE FOODS	473		7.5	51.2	26.8
sweet chilli KETTLE FOODS	466		7.1	53	25.4
Kettle Vegetables					
golden parsnip KETTLE FOODS	515		4.6	39.5	37.6
select vegetables KETTLE FOODS	487		5.5	39.2	34.2
sweet potato KETTLE FOODS	483		2.4	44.4	32.8
Limbos					
cheese & onion RYVITA	352		12.1	69.1	3
salt & vinegar RYVITA	344		9.8	72	1.9
smokey bacon RYVITA	352		14.3	69.7	1.8

Food Type	cal per 100g	cal per portion	pro (g)	carb (g)	fat (g)
Pickled Onion Crisps					
per pack (34.5g) GOLDENWONDER		178	1.8	18.5	10.7
Potato Crisps	530		5.7	53.3	34.2
low-fat	458		6.6	63.5	21.5
Prawn Cocktail Crisps					
per pack (34.5g) GOLDENWONDER		179	1.9	18.7	10.7
Pringles					
PROCTOR & GAMBLE	540		4.1	49	36
cheesy cheese PROCTOR & GAMBLE	534		5	48	35
cheese & onion PROCTOR & GAMBLE	528		4.1	50	34
hot & spicy PROCTOR & GAMBLE	530		4.6	49	34
paprika PROCTOR & GAMBLE	529		49	3.2	34
prawn cocktail PROCTOR & GAMBLE	528		4.9	49	34
salt & vinegar PROCTOR & GAMBLE	527		3.9	50	34
smokey bacon PROCTOR & GAMBLE	551		5.1	49	34
sour cream & onion					
PROCTOR & GAMBLE	527		3.9	50	34
Texas BBQ sauce PROCTOR &					
GAMBLE	527		4.2	50	34
Pringles Light Aromas					
PROCTOR & GAMBLE	484		4.3	59	25
Greek style cheese					
PROCTOR & GAMBLE	488		4.6	57	25
Mediterranean style salsa					
PROCTOR & GAMBLE	472		4.7	58	25

Food Type	cal per 100g	cal per portion	pro (g)	carb (g)	fat (g)
red pepper PROCTOR & GAMBLE	482		4.6	58	24
sour cream & onion					
PROCTOR & GAMBLE	487		4.7	57	25
spicy Thai PROCTOR & GAMBLE	485		4.1	59	24
Quavers					
cheese, per pack (16.4g) WALKERS		87	0.4	10.2	4.9
Ready Salted Crisps					
per pack (34.5g) GOLDENWONDER		180	1.7	18.1	11.2
per pack (34.5g) WALKERS		183	n/a	n/a	11.7
Baked, per pack (25g) WALKERS		98	1.5	18.5	2
Lights, per pack (24g) WALKERS		113	1.7	14.6	5.3
Rice Infusions					
cheese & onion PROCTOR & GAMBLE	487		5.2	60	24
hot & spicy PROCTOR & GAMBLE	530		4.6	49	34
Peking duck PROCTOR & GAMBLE	490		5.4	60	24
red paprika PROCTOR & GAMBLE	487		5.2	60	24
salt & vinegar PROCTOR & GAMBLE	486		4.8	60	24
sour cream & onion					
PROCTOR & GAMBLE	493		5.3	59	24
sweet BBQ spare rib					
PROCTOR & GAMBLE	487		4.8	60	24
sweet & sour PROCTOR & GAMBLE	491		4.7	61	24
Thai chilli & lime PROCTOR & GAMBLE	488		4.9	60	24
Ringos					
cheese & onion, per pack (34g)					
GOLDENWONDER		81	1.2	11.6	3.3

Food Type	cal per 100g	cal per portion	pro (g)	carb (g)	fat (g)
pickled onion, per pack (34g)					
GOLDENWONDER		79	1	11.3	3.3
salt & vinegar, per pack (34g)					
GOLDENWONDER		79	1	11.4	3.3
Roast Chicken Crisps					
per pack (34.5g) GOLDENWONDER		178	1.9	18.4	10.7
Salt & Vinegar Crisps					
per pack (34.5g) GOLDENWONDER		176	1.7	18.1	10.7
per pack (34.5g) WALKERS		181	2.2	17.3	11.4
baked, per pack (25g) WALKERS		98	1.5	18.3	2
Salt & Vinegar Golden Lights					
per pack (21g) GOLDENWONDER		93	0.9	13.7	3.8
Sausage & Tomato Crisps					
per pack (34.5g) GOLDENWONDER		178	1.9	18.5	10.7
Sea Salt Golden Lights					
per pack (21g) GOLDENWONDER		94	0.9	13.6	4
Sensations					
balsamic vinegar & onion WALKERS	485		6.1	57	26
buffalo mozzarella & herb WALKERS	490		6.1	57	26
chicken & thyme WALKERS	485		6	56	26
oriental red curry WALKERS	485		6	57	26
Southern style BBQ WALKERS	485		6.3	57	26
Thai sweet chilli WALKERS	485		6	57	26
vintage cheddar & chutney					
WALKERS	480		6.3	58	25

Food Type	cal per 100g	cal per portion	pro (g)	carb (g)	fat (g)
Skips					
prawn cocktail, per pack (17g)					
UNITED BISCUITS		89	1.1	9.9	5
sizzling bacon, per pack (17g)					
UNITED BISCUITS		89	1.2	9.9	5
utterly cheesy, per pack (17g)					
UNITED BISCUITS		89	1.2	9.8	5
Smokey Bacon Crisps					
per pack (34.5g) GOLDENWONDER		178	1.9	18.4	10.7
Sour Cream & Chive Crisps					
lights, per pack (24g) WALKERS		114	1.8	14.9	5.3
Sour Cream & Onion					
Golden Lights					
per pack (21g) GOLDENWONDER		94	1	13.6	3.9
Spring Onion Crisps					
per pack (34.5g) GOLDENWONDER		177	1.8	18.4	10.7
Squares					
cheese & onion, per pack (22g)					
WALKERS		95	1.4	13.4	4
ready salted, per pack (22g)					
WALKERS		96	1.4	13.2	4.2
salt & vinegar, per pack (22g)					
WALKERS		95	1.4	13.4	4
Tomato Ketchup Crisps					
per pack (34.5g) GOLDENWONDER		178	1.8	18.5	10.7

Food Type	cal per 100g	cal per portion	pro (g)	carb (g)	fat (g)
Wheat Crunchies					
big cheese, per pack (30g)					
UNITED BISCUITS		151	2.9	16.4	8.2
crispy bacon, per pack (25g)					
UNITED BISCUITS		126	2.3	13.9	6.8
spicy tomato, per pack (25g)					
UNITED BISCUITS		126	2.3	14	6.7
Worcester sauce, per pack (25g)					
UNITED BISCUITS		126	2.2	14	6.7
Wotsits					
flamin' hot, per pack (19g)					
WALKERS		93	1	10.5	5.3
prawn cocktail, per pack (19g)					
WALKERS		91	0.8	10.2	5.3
really cheesy, per pack (19g)					
WALKERS		104	1	10.6	6.3
Nibbles					
Bombay Mix					
JULIAN GRAVES	479		18.9	25.5	33.5
Bruschettine					
with basil & parmesan BERTOLLLI	424		11.8	73.3	11
with rosemary & sea salt BERTOLLLI	419		11.1	71.8	11.5
Cashews					
salted	615		20	19	51
roasted, salted JULIAN GRAVES	615		20.5	18.8	50.9

Food Type	cal per 100g	cal per portion	pro (g)	carb (g)	fat (g)
Cheese Flavoured Puffs					
WEIGHTWATCHERS	417		7.8	72.4	10.8
Cheese Oat Bakes					
NAIRN	422		14.6	60.5	13.6
Cheeselets					
JACOB'S	492		9.8	55.5	25.7
Cheez Dippers					
FROMAGERIES BEL	288		11	25	16
Collisions					
chicken sizzler & zesty salsa					
DORITOS	492		6.7	59.6	25.2
t-bone steak & grilled pepper					
DORITOS	489		6.5	59.2	25.2
Doritos					
chilli heatwave WALKERS	500		7	60	26
cool original WALKERS	500		7.5	58	27
hint of lime WALKERS	510		6.5	60	27
lightly salted WALKERS	510		6.5	60	27
tangy cheese WALKERS	500		8.2	57.1	26.5
Focaccine with parsley & garlic					
BERTOLLLI	446	9.9	10.1	67.2	16.7
Focaccine with tomato & oregano					
BERTOLLLI	446	9.9	66.8	16.9	11.5

Food Type	cal per 100g	cal per portion	pro (g)	carb (g)	fat (g)
Macadamia Nuts					
salted	748		7.9	4.8	77.6
roasted & salted JULIAN GRAVES	767		7.8	12.8	76.1
Mediterranean Tomato Oat Bakes					
NAIRN	431		8.1	64.2	15.8
Minis					
cream cheese & chives RYVITA	342		8	71	2.9
mature cheddar & onion RYVITA	337		9.3	68.2	3
salt & vinegar RYVITA	312		6.8	64.8	2.8
sweet chilli RYVITA	335		7	71	2.6
Thai RYVITA	334		8.1	70.4	2.2
Worcester sauce RYVITA	339		6.9	71.9	2.6
Mini Bagels					
cream cheeese & chive,					
per pack (35g) SNACK-A-JACK		145	3.7	25	3.4
Mini Cheddars					
MCVITIES	516		11.2	50.7	29.8
Nachips					
OLD EL PASO	506		7	61	26
Nik Naks					
cream 'n' cheesy, per pack (25g)					
UNITED BISCUITS		141	1.3	12.4	9.6
nice 'n' spicy, per pack (25g)					
UNITED BISCUITS		140	1.2	12.4	9.6

Food Type	cal per 100g	cal per portion	pro (g)	carb (g)	fat (g)
pickle 'n' onion, per pack (30g)					
UNITED BISCUITS		170	1.5	15.1	11.5
rib 'n' saucy, per pack (25g)					
UNITED BISCUITS		141	1.3	12.5	9.6
scampi 'n' lemon, per					
pack (25g) UNITED BISCUITS		141	1.3	12.4	9.6
Oat Bites, Mild Chilli					
PATERSON'S	447		13.2	53.3	20.1
Peanuts					
dry roasted	590		25.7	10.3	49.8
roasted & salted	602		24.7	7.1	53
blanched JULIAN GRAVES	611		25.8	16.1	49.2
dry roasted JULIAN GRAVES	583		23.4	13	48.6
salted JULIAN GRAVES	631		25.6	8.4	55
Peanuts & Raisins	436		15.4	37.5	25.9
yogurt-coated HOLLAND & BARRETT	465		8.9	54.3	25.8
Pepite with Italian Cheese & Red Onion					
BERTOLLLI	464	9.9	8.9	64	20.4
Pistachio Nuts					
roasted & salted	599		18	8	55
roasted & salted JULIAN GRAVES	606		21.4	26.8	46
Popcorn	593		6.2	48.7	42.8
Butter Toffee SNACK-A-JACK	425		3.5	86	9
Candied	480		2.1	77.6	20

Food Type	cal per 100g	cal per portion	pro (g)	carb (g)	fat (g)
Chocolate SNACK-A-JACK	359		2.2	65	9.8
Lightly Salted SNACK-A-JACK	370		12	58	9.9
Salt & Vinegar SNACK-A-JACK	360		12	55	9.9
Uncooked CYPRESSA	592		6.2	48.6	42.8
Pappadums					
fried in vegetable oil	369		17.5	39.1	16.9
Cook to Eat SHARWOOD	273		21.9	45.7	0.3
Garlic & Coriander, ready to eat					
PATAK	434		19.2	43.9	21.5
Garlic & Coriander, ready to eat					
SHARWOOD	438		18.4	43	21.4
Plain, ready to eat PATAK	415		19.4	43.4	18.6
Plain, ready to eat SHARWOOD	461		19.4	46.3	22
Pappadums, Mini					
Chilli & Lime, ready to eat					
PATAK	470		14.6	42	27.1
Mint Raita, ready to eat PATAK	477		15.7	41.2	27.7
Pecans					
yogurt-flavoured coated					
JULIAN GRAVES	580		5.4	44.7	42.2
Prawn Crackers					
ready to eat BLUE DRAGON	508		3.4	56	30
ready to eat SHARWOOD	520		1.3	60.2	30.4
Rice Crackers					
BLUE DRAGON	376		7	79.7	3.2

Food Type	cal per 100g	cal per portion	pro (g)	carb (g)	fat (g)
cheese BLUE DRAGON	379		7.3	79	3.7
chilli BLUE DRAGON	377		6.9	80.1	3.2
Snack					
each, Philadelphia KRAFT		117	4.4	12	5.7
Snack-a-Jacks Jumbo					
barbecue PEPSICO	380		8	83	2
caramel flavour PEPSICO	390		5.5	87	2.1
cheese flavour PEPSICO	380		8.5	81	2.5
salt & vinegar PEPSICO	172		7.4	74.5	5.7
Snack-a-Jacks Snacks					
barbecue, per pack (30g) PEPSICO		123	2.3	24	1.8
caramel, per pack (35g) PEPSICO		142	2.1	30.8	1.1
cheese, per pack (30g) PEPSICO		125	2.6	23	2.4
prawn cocktail, per pack (30g) PEPSICO		123	2.1	23.4	2.3
salt & vinegar, per pack (30g) PEPSICO		123	2.1	23.7	2.3
sour cream & chive, per pack (30g) PEPSICO		125	2.4	23.7	2.3
Snack-a-Jacks Mini Bites					
mature cheddar & red onion, per pack (28g) PEPSICO		116	2.1	21.3	2.5
sour cream & sweet chilli, per pack (28g) PEPSICO		115	1.8	21.8	2.2

Food Type	cal per 100g	cal per portion	pro (g)	carb (g)	fat (g)
Sunbites					
per pack (25g) WALKERS		118	1.8	15.1	5.6
roasted onion & rosemary,					
per pack (25g) WALKERS		117	1.9	15.1	5.4
sour cream & cracked black					
pepper, per pack (25g) WALKERS		117	1.9	15.1	5.4
sun-ripened sweet chilli,					
per pack (25g) WALKERS		117	1.8	15.3	5.4
Sweet Chillli Oat Bakes					
NAIRN	426		8.1	68.4	13.3
Thai Spiced Crackers					
SHARWOOD	515		1.2	68.7	26.2
Tomato Oat Bakes					
NAIRN	431		8.1	64.2	15.8
Tortilla Chips	459		7.6	60.1	22.6
all varieties HULA HOOPS	494		4.9	57.2	27.3
Sour Cream & Mexican Chilli					
PHILEAS FOGG	489		5.2	60.4	25.1
Salsa with Mexican Chilli					
PHILEAS FOGG	489		5.4	60.2	25.2
Trail Mix	415		2.8	44.8	24.8
Twiglets					
original JACOB'S	383		12.7	57	11.6

Food Type

	cal per 100g	cal per portion	pro (g)	carb (g)	fat (g)
Dairy					
Milk & Cream					
Buttermilk					
cultured, pasturised	66		6.3	9.7	0.2
Cream					
fresh, clotted	586		1.6	2.3	63.5
fresh, double	496		1.6	1.7	53.7
fresh, extra thick	445		1.7	2.6	47.5
fresh, half	162		2.7	4.4	15
fresh, single	193		3.3	2.2	19.1
fresh, soured	205		2.9	3.8	19.9
fresh, whipping	381		2	2.7	40.3
sterilised, canned	239		2.5	3.7	23.9
UHT, aerosol spray	252		1.9	7.2	24.2
Crème Fraîche					
full fat	378		2.2	2.4	40
half fat	162		2.7	4.4	15
Milk, fresh					
cows', whole, average	66		3.3	4.5	3.9
cows', semi-skimmed, average	46		3.4	4.7	1.7
cows', skimmed, average	32		3.4	4.4	0.2
cows', Channel Island	78		3.6	4.8	5.1
goats', pasteurised	62		3.1	4.4	3.7
sheep's, raw	93		5.4	5.1	5.8

Food Type	cal per 100g	cal per portion	pro (g)	carb (g)	fat (g)
Milk, dried					
skimmed	348		36.1	52.9	0.6
Milk, condensed					
whole milk, sweetened	333		8.5	55.5	10.1
skimmed milk, sweetened	267		10	60	0.2
Cream					
extra thick, aerosol ANCHOR	93		0.4	0.4	9.9
fresh, single, organic YEO VALLEY	193		3.3	2.2	19.1
fresh, double, organic YEO VALLEY	459		1.7	2.8	49
fresh, extra thick, organic					
YEO VALLEY	294		2.3	3.6	30
UHT, cream swirls (aerosol)					
ANCHOR	66		0.4	1.4	6.5
UHT, single ELMLEA	148		3.1	4.6	13
UHT, single, light ELMLEA	117		3.1	4.8	9.5
UHT, double ELMLEA	349		2.4	3.9	36
UHT, double, light ELMLEA	231		2.5	3.5	23
UHT, whipping ELMLEA	290		2.4	3.6	29.6
Crème Fraîche					
organic YEO VALLEY	179		2.6	3.7	17.1
Milk, fresh					
cows', whole, organic YEO VALLEY	68		3.4	4	4
cows', semi-skimmed, organic					
YEO VALLEY	47		3.6	4.8	1.8

Dairy

Food Type	cal per 100g	cal per portion	pro (g)	carb (g)	fat (g)
cows', skimmed, organic					
YEO VALLEY	35		3.6	4.9	0.3
goats', whole ST HELEN'S FARM	61		2.8	4.3	3.6
goats', semi-skimmed					
ST HELEN'S FARM	44		3	4.3	1.6
goats', skimmed ST HELEN'S FARM	30		3	4.3	0.1
Milk, condensed					
Carnation NESTLÉ	330		8.3	54.3	9.1
Carnation Caramel NESTLÉ	296		5.5	55	6
Carnation Light NESTLÉ	289		10	60.4	0.2
Milk, evaporated					
Carnation NESTLÉ	162		7.7	12.4	9
Carnation Light NESTLÉ	110		6.9	11.3	4
Milk, dried					
skimmed, as sold MARVEL	361		36.1	52.9	0.6
made up with water MARVEL	206		20.6	30.2	0.3
Yogurt & Fromage Frais					
Non-branded Yogurt					
Greek-style, cows', fruit	137		4.8	11.2	8.4
Greek-style, cows', plain	133		5.7	4.8	10.2
Greek-style, sheep's	92		4.8	5	6
low-fat, fruit	78		4.2	13.7	1.1
low-fat, plain	56		4.8	7.4	1
soya, fruit	73		2.1	12.9	1.8

Food Type	cal per 100g	cal per portion	pro (g)	carb (g)	fat (g)
virtually fat-free, fruit	47		4.8	7	0.2
virtually fat-free, plain	54		5.4	8.2	0.2
whole milk, fruit	109		4	17.7	3
whole milk, plain	79		5.7	7.8	3
Non-branded Fromage Frais					
fruit	124		5.3	13.9	5.6
plain	113		6.1	4.4	8
virtually fat-free, fruit	50		6.8	5.6	0.2
virtually fat-free, plain	49		7.7	4.6	0.1
Activia Fibre					
cereals DANONE	100		3.9	13.5	3.4
kiwi cereals DANONE	103		3.8	14.5	3.3
Activia Fruit Layer					
blueberry & blackberry DANONE	86		3.3	11.7	2.9
prune DANONE	83		3.2	11.3	2.8
raspberry DANONE	80		3.2	10.5	2.8
Activia Intensely Creamy					
luscious cherry DANONE	97		4.8	12.7	3
peaches & cream DANONE	98		4.8	13	3
sumptuous strawberry DANONE	97		4.8	12.8	3
zesty lemon DANONE	99		4.8	13.3	3
Amoré Luxury Yogurts					
cherry indulgent MÜLLER	143		2.6	16.8	7.3
orange indulgent MÜLLER	145		2.7	17.1	7.3

Food Type	cal per 100g	cal per portion	pro (g)	carb (g)	fat (g)
peach indulgent MÜLLER	144		2.6	17	7.3
strawberry indulgent MÜLLER	144		2.6	17	7.3
vanilla & dark chocolate flake indulgent MÜLLER	170		2.7	18.4	9.5
walnut & greek honey indulgent MÜLLER	160		3	17.4	8.7
Apricot Flavour Pro.active Yogurt					
FLORA	56		4	7.9	0.5
Apricot Whole Milk Yogurt					
organic YEO VALLEY	98		4.3	11.7	3.7
Apricot Yogurt					
low fat SKI	73		4.5	13.6	0.1
Black Cherry Yogurt					
SKI	97		4.3	16.1	1.7
Blackberry Fromage Frais					
WEIGHTWATCHERS	64		5.3	10.4	0.2
Blackberry Yogurt					
SHAPE	61		6.7	8.4	0.1
Blueberry Yogurt					
SHAPE	63		6.7	8.8	0.1
fat-free, organic YEO VALLEY	73		5.1	12.9	0.1
whole milk, organic YEO VALLEY	95		4.2	11.7	3.5
Cherry Fromage Frais					
WEIGHTWATCHERS	64		5.3	10.8	0.1

Food Type	cal per 100g	cal per portion	pro (g)	carb (g)	fat (g)
Cherry Yogurt					
ONKEN	108		3.8	16.9	2.7
SHAPE	62		6.6	8.7	0.1
fat-free ACTIVIA	57		4.7	9.4	0.1
low-fat, organic YEO VALLEY	83		5.1	13.2	1
Exotic Fruit Yogurt					
SHAPE	65		6.6	8.7	0.1
Forest Fruit Yogurt					
fat-free ACTIVIA	54		4.7	8.6	0.1
Forest Fruits Fromage Frais					
WEIGHTWATCHERS	62		5.5	9.6	0.2
Fruit Corner					
blackberry & raspberry MÜLLER	106		3.8	13.2	3.9
blueberry MÜLLER	105		3.8	12.9	3.9
cherry MÜLLER	106		3.8	13.2	3.9
peach & apricot MÜLLER	108		3.8	13.7	3.9
strawberry MÜLLER	113		3.8	14.9	3.9
Fruit of the Forest Yogurt					
SHAPE	62		6.7	8.5	0.1
Goats' Milk Yogurt					
natural ST HELEN'S FARM	105		5.5	4.3	7.3
Greek Style Yogurt					
honey, organic YEO VALLEY	154		4.1	15.2	8.5
natural, organic YEO VALLEY	136		4.7	6.9	10
strawberry, organic YEO VALLEY	147		4.2	13.3	8.5

Food Type	cal per 100g	cal per portion	pro (g)	carb (g)	fat (g)
Lemon Yogurt					
fat-free WEIGHTWATCHERS	41		4	5.8	0.1
fat-free organic YEO VALLEY	82		5	15.4	0.1
Lemon & Lime Yogurt					
fat-free WEIGHTWATCHERS	41		4.1	5.9	0.1
Mango Yogurt					
SHAPE	62		6.6	8.6	0.1
Mango, Papaya & Passion Fruit Yogurt					
ONKEN	104		3.8	15.8	2.7
Mango & Passion Fruit Yogurt					
organic YEO VALLEY	114		5.1	13.6	4.3
Mango & Passionfruit Tropical Yogurt					
SKI	95		4.3	15.6	1.7
Mixed Berry Yogurt					
organic YEO VALLEY	96		4.2	11.8	3.6
Müllerlight					
banana & custard yogurt MÜLLER	53		4	8.4	0.1
blackcurrant yogurt MÜLLER	50		4.1	7.6	0.1
blackcurrant & raspberry layers yogurt MÜLLER	54		3.1	9.6	0.1
cherry yogurt MÜLLER	47		4.1	6.7	0.1
chocolate yogurt MÜLLER	51		4	7.1	0.5
mandarin yogurt MÜLLER	52		4	8.2	0.1

Food Type	cal per 100g	cal per portion	pro (g)	carb (g)	fat (g)
peach yogurt MÜLLER	47		4.1	6.9	0.1
peach & pineapple yogurt MÜLLER	49		4.1	7.4	0.1
raspberry & cranberry yogurt MÜLLER	50		4.1	7.6	0.1
rhubarb yogurt MÜLLER	50		4.1	7.6	0.1
strawberry layers yogurt MÜLLER	54		3.1	9.6	0.1
strawberry yogurt MÜLLER	51		4.1	7.7	0.1
toffee yogurt MÜLLER	50		4	7.7	0.1
vanilla yogurt MÜLLER	50		4.3	7.2	0.1
vanilla & chocolate MÜLLER	52		4	7.2	0.5
wild blueberry yogurt MÜLLER	47		4.1	6.9	0.1
Munch Bunch Fromage Frais					
apricot NESTLÉ	106		6	13.1	3.1
raspberry NESTLÉ	104		6	12.8	3.1
strawberry NESTLÉ	104		6	12.8	3.1
Munch Bunch Wholemilk Yogurt					
banana NESTLÉ	98		3.5	13.6	3
blackcurrant & apple NESTLÉ	99		3.6	13.6	3
raspberry NESTLÉ	99		3.6	13.6	3
strawberry NESTLÉ	98		3.5	13.5	3
Natural Yogurt					
ACTIVIA	61		4.9	6.1	1.9
smooth ONKEN	78		5	6.1	3.7
whole milk, organic YEO VALLEY	82		4.5	6.6	4.2

Food Type	cal per 100g	cal per portion	pro (g)	carb (g)	fat (g)
Orange & Nectarine Yogurt					
fat-free WEIGHTWATCHERS	41		4.1	6	0.1
Peach Yogurt					
fat-free ACTIVIA	57		4.7	9.3	0.1
fat-free SKI	74		4.5	13.7	0.1
low-fat, organic YEO VALLEY	82		5.1	13.1	1
with wholegrains ONKEN	114		4.2	18	2.8
Peach & Passionfruit Tropical Yogurt					
SKI	92		4.3	15	1.7
Peach & Passionfruit Yogurt					
SHAPE	62		6.6	8.1	0.1
Petits Filous Fromage Frais					
YOPLAIT	104		6.6	12.6	2.9
Petits Filous Frubes					
YOPLAIT	110		6.7	14.1	2.9
Pineapple Yogurt					
SHAPE	62		6.6	8.7	0.1
Pink Grapefruit Yogurt					
fat-free WEIGHTWATCHERS	41		3.9	6.2	0.1
Prune Flavour Pro.active Yogurt					
FLORA	57		4.1	8.1	0.5
Raspberry Flavour Pro.active Yogurt					
FLORA	54		4.1	7.4	0.5

Food Type	cal per 100g	cal per portion	pro (g)	carb (g)	fat (g)
Raspberry Fromage Frais					
WEIGHTWATCHERS	51		5.5	6.3	0.1
Raspberry Whole Milk Yogurt					
organic YEO VALLEY	98		4.3	11.6	3.7
Raspberry Yogurt					
ONKEN	102		3.9	15.2	2.7
SHAPE	61		6.7	8.4	0.1
fat-free ACTIVIA	47		4.6	6.9	0.1
fat-free SKI	76		4.6	14.1	0.1
fat-free, organic YEO VALLEY	75		5.3	13	0.1
smooth SKI	94		4.6	14.8	1.7
Raspberry & Cranberry Yogurt					
whole milk, organic YEO VALLEY	96		4.3	11.7	3.5
Red Cherry Yogurt					
SKI	96		4.3	15.8	1.7
Rhubarb Yogurt					
fat-free, organic YEO VALLEY	71		5.1	12.4	0.1
low-fat, organic YEO VALLEY	79		5.1	12.4	1
Rhubarb & Vanilla Yogurt					
ONKEN	107		3.8	16.7	2.7
Strawberry Flavour Pro.active Yogurt					
FLORA	54		4.1	7.5	0.5
Strawberry Whole Milk Yogurt					
organic YEO VALLEY	99		4.3	11.8	3.7

Food Type	cal per 100g	cal per portion	pro (g)	carb (g)	fat (g)
Strawberry Yogurt					
SHAPE	60		6.6	8.2	0.1
fat-free ONKEN	55		4.9	8.1	0.1
fat-free SKI	74		4.5	13.7	0.2
fat-free, organic YEO VALLEY	75		5.3	13.2	0.1
low-fat, organic YEO VALLEY	82		5.1	13.1	1
smooth SKI	94		4.6	14.8	1.7
with wholegrains ONKEN	114		4.2	17.4	2.9
Strawberry & Raspberry Smoothies Yogurt					
organic YEO VALLEY	98		4.3	11.7	3.7
Strawberry & Redcurrant Yogurt					
whole milk, organic YEO VALLEY	96		4.3	11.8	3.5
Strawberry & Vanilla Smoothies Yogurt					
organic YEO VALLEY	99		4.3	11.8	3.7
Summer Berries Yogurt					
with wholegrains ONKEN	111		4.2	17.1	2.9
Summer Fruits Layers, low fat					
apricot WEIGHTWATCHERS	58		5.4	8.1	0.1
peach WEIGHTWATCHERS	57		5.4	7.9	0.1
raspberry WEIGHTWATCHERS	51		5.5	6.3	0.1
strawberry WEIGHTWATCHERS	50		5.4	6.2	0.1
Toffee Flavour Yogurts					
fat-free WEIGHTWATCHERS	40		3.9	5.9	0.1

Food Type	cal per 100g	cal per portion	pro (g)	carb (g)	fat (g)
Toffee Fromage Frais					
WEIGHTWATCHERS	59		5.2	9.3	0.1
Toffee Yogurt					
low fat, organic YEO VALLEY	88		5.4	14.3	1
Vanilla Flavour Yogurt					
fat-free WEIGHTWATCHERS	40		3.9	5.9	0.1
Vanilla Yogurt					
fat-free ACTIVIA	52		4.9	7.8	0.1
fat-free, organic YEO VALLEY	80		5.4	14.2	0.1
Very Berry Yogurt					
blackberry SKI	95		4.4	15.5	1.7
loganberry SKI	93		4.4	15.1	1.7
raspberry SKI	95		4.4	15.5	1.7
strawberry SKI	92		4.3	15	1.7
Vitality					
apricot MÜLLER	90		4.3	13.6	1.7
blackcurrant MÜLLER	91		4.3	14	1.7
blueberry MÜLLER	93		4.2	13.7	1.7
cherry MÜLLER	94		4.3	14.7	1.7
peach & passionfruit MÜLLER	91		4.3	14	1.7
raspberry MÜLLER	91		4.3	13.6	1.8
red berry MÜLLER	92		4.3	14.2	1.7
strawberry MÜLLER	91		4.3	13.8	1.7
Wildlife Fromage Frais					
YOPLAIT	109		6.4	14.1	3

Dairy

Food Type

Food Type	cal per 100g	cal per portion	pro (g)	carb (g)	fat (g)
Yogurt Drinks					
Actimel					
DANONE	72		3	10.5	1.6
blueberry DANONE	76		2.9	11.8	1.5
cherry DANONE	74		2.9	11.5	1.5
coconut DANONE	80		2.9	11.9	1.9
forest fruits DANONE	74		2.9	11.5	1.5
low fat DANONE	28		2.8	3.3	0.1
low fat, peach & mango DANONE	29		2.7	3.6	0.1
low fat, raspberry DANONE	29		2.7	3.7	0.1
low fat, strawberry DANONE	29		2.7	3.7	0.1
multifruit DANONE	76		2.9	12	1.5
orange DANONE	74		2.9	11.5	1.5
strawberry DANONE	74		2.9	11.5	1.5
vanilla DANONE	78		2.9	12.5	1.5
Benecol Yogurt Drink					
each MCNEIL CONSUMER NUTRITIONAL	61		1.8	10	1.5
light, each MCNEIL CONSUMER NUTRITIONAL	41		1.9	5	1.5
strawberry, each MCNEIL CONSUMER NUTRITIONAL	39		2.2	4.3	1.5
Pro.active Yogurt Drinks, all flavours FLORA	87		2.6	12.5	2.9
Vitality Drink					
blueberry, each MÜLLER		66	2.6	10.3	1.4

Food Type	cal per 100g	cal per portion	pro (g)	carb (g)	fat (g)
mango, *each MÜLLER*		66	2.6	10.3	1.4
peach, *each MÜLLER*		70	2.5	11.3	1.4
raspberry, *each MÜLLER*		68	2.5	10.9	1.4
strawberry, *each MÜLLER*		67	2.5	10.7	1.4
vanilla, *each MÜLLER*		70	2.4	11.5	1.4
Yakult Fermented Milk Drink					
YAKULT UK	74		1.4	17.2	Tr
light YAKULT UK	42		1.4	10.2	Tr
Yogurt, Oats, Raspberries & Blueberries					
thickie, *each INNOCENT*		223	11	41.8	3.5
Yogurt, Vanilla Bean & Honey					
thickie, *each INNOCENT*		230	10.8	41.3	2.8
Yop					
raspberry YOPLAIT	77		2.8	13.4	1.3
strawberry YOPLAIT	78		2.8	13.4	1.3
Butter & Margarines					
Butter					
salted & unsalted	744		0.6	0.6	82.2
spreadable	745		0.5	Tr	82.5
Margarine, hard					
animal & vegetable fat, over 80% fat	718		0.2	1	79.3
Margarine, soft					
polyunsaturated, over 80% fat	746		Tr	0.2	82.8

Dairy

209

Food Type	cal per 100g	cal per portion	pro (g)	carb (g)	fat (g)
Butter					
lighter, spreadable LURPAK	544		0.5	0.5	60
lightly salted ANCHOR	750		0.6	0.6	82.8
lightly salted LURPAK	742		1	1	81.5
lightly salted, organic YEO VALLEY	737		0.5	Tr	81.7
lightly salted, spreadable LURPAK	728		1	1	80
spreadable, organic LURPAK	728		1	1	80
spreadable, organic YEO VALLEY	720		0.4	0.5	80
unsalted ANCHOR	750		0.6	0.6	82.8
unsalted LURPAK	749		0	0.8	82.4
unsalted, organic YEO VALLEY	752		0.6	0.8	82.9
unsalted, spreadable LURPAK	726		1	0.5	80
with garlic LURPAK	695		1	4	75
Stork					
block STORK	675		0	0	75
tub STORK	531		Tr	Tr	59
Spreads					
Benecol					
buttery BENECOL	572		0.3	0.5	53
light BENECOL	329		2.8	0.2	35
olive BENECOL	498		0.3	0.5	55
Bertolli					
olive oil spread BERTOLLI	536		0.2	1	59
olive oil spread, light BERTOLLI	353		Tr	2.5	38

Food Type	cal per 100g	cal per portion	pro (g)	carb (g)	fat (g)
Clover					
DAIRY CREST	681		0.6	0.8	75
lighter DAIRY CREST	455		0.7	2.9	49
Flora					
buttery FLORA	532		Tr	0.2	59
extra light FLORA	227		3.5	1.6	23
light FLORA	366		0.1	6	38
no salt FLORA	531		Tr	Tr	59
omega 3 plus FLORA	350		0.1	3	38
original FLORA	531		Tr	Tr	59
pro.active FLORA	331		0.1	4	35
pro.active with olive oil FLORA	331		0.1	4	35
I Can't Believe It's Not Butter					
UNILEVER	635		0.5	0.7	70
Utterly Butterly					
ST IVEL	534		0.3	0.5	59
Cheeses					
Babybel					
mini FROMAGERIES BEL	315		22.5	0.1	25
Babybel Cheddar					
mini FROMAGERIES BEL	362		23	0.1	30
Babybel Light					
mini FROMAGERIES BEL	210		25.5	0.1	12

Food Type	cal per 100g	cal per portion	pro (g)	carb (g)	fat (g)
Bavarian Smoked	277		17	0.4	23
Boursin					
garlic & herbs BOURSIN	405		7	2	41
garlic & herbs, light BOURSIN	140		12	2.5	9
Brie	305		22	0.5	24
COEUR DE LION	322		17	0.5	28
Caerphilly	371		23	0.1	31
Cambozola	430		13	0.5	42
Camembert	290		21.5	Tr	22.7
Cathedral City					
DAIRY CREST	416		25.4	0.1	34.9
lighter DAIRY CREST	311		28.6	0.1	21.8
Cheddar					
extra mature, organic YEO VALLEY	410		25	0.1	34.4
mature, low fat WEIGHT WATCHERS	217		31	0.1	10.3
mature, organic YEO VALLEY	410		25	0.1	34.4
medium, organic YEO VALLEY	410		25	0.1	34.4
Cheddar-type, half fat	273		32.7	Tr	15.8
Cheshire	371		23	0.1	31
organic YEO VALLEY	377		23.5	0.1	31.4
Cottage Cheese					
plain	101		12.6	3.1	4.3
natural	120		12	3.6	6
reduced fat	79		13.3	3.3	1.5

Food Type	cal per 100g	cal per portion	pro (g)	carb (g)	fat (g)
reduced fat, with onion & chive	79		12	4.4	1.5
reduced fat, with pineapple	85		9	10	1
Cracker Barrel Cheddar					
KRAFT	395		26	0.1	32
Cream Cheese	439		3.1	Tr	47.4
Danish Blue	342		20.5	Tr	28.9
Dolcelatte	395		17	0.8	36
Double Gloucester	402		24	0.1	34
organic YEO VALLEY	404		24.4	0.1	34
Edam	341		26.7	Tr	26
Emmenthal	370		29	0.4	28
Feta	250		15.6	1.5	20.2
Goats' Milk Soft Cheese	320		21.1	1	25.8
Gorgonzola	310		19	0	26
Gouda	377		25.3	Tr	30.6
Grana Padano	392		35	0	28
Gruyère	396		27	0.1	32
Jarlsberg	364		28	0	28
TINE	351		27	Tr	27
Lancashire	371		23	0.1	31
Laughing Cow					
FROMAGERIES BEL	269		10	6.5	22.5
light FROMAGERIES BEL	141		13	6.5	7

Dairy

Food Type	cal per 100g	cal per portion	pro (g)	carb (g)	fat (g)
Mascarpone	416		4.8	4.8	42
organic BRESCIA	451		4.8	2.2	47
Medium Fat Soft Cheese	199		9.8	3.5	16.3
Mozzarella	240		18	1.5	18
DISCOVER	303		26	1	21.7
organic BRESCIA	262		18.1	1.5	20.4
Santa Lucia GALBANI	247		18	1	19
Parmesan, fresh	415		36.2	0.9	29.7
Parmesan, fresh, grated	384		33	0.9	28
Parmesan, dried, grated					
NAPOLINA	490		45	0	34
Philadelphia Soft Cheese					
extra light KRAFT	111		12	5	4.7
full fat KRAFT	255		5.9	3.2	24
light, medium fat KRAFT	155		8.2	4.1	11.5
light, with basil KRAFT	146		8	4	10.5
light, with chives KRAFT	160		8.4	4.2	12
light, with garlic & herbs KRAFT	156		8.2	3.9	11.5
Quark	61		11	3.9	0.2
Red Leicester	402		24	0.1	34
organic YEO VALLEY	399		23.8	0.1	33.7
Reduced Fat Mature Cheese					
WEIGHTWATCHERS	188		36.1	6	2.3

Food Type	cal per 100g	cal per portion	pro (g)	carb (g)	fat (g)
Ricotta	134		9	2	10
organic BRESCIA	126		9	3.5	9.5
Roquefort	355		23	Tr	29.2
Sage Derby	415		24.4	2.7	34
Shropshire Blue	369		22	0.5	31
Soft Cheese with Roasted Onion & Chive					
WEIGHTWATCHERS	95		12.9	5.1	2.5
Stilton					
blue	410		23.7	0.1	35
white	359		20	0.1	31
white, with apricots	321		16	8	25
Wensleydale	380		23	0.1	32
with cranberries	363		21	9	27
Cheese Spreads & Processed Cheese					
Cheese Spread					
plain	267		11.3	4.4	22.8
reduced fat	175		15	7.9	9.5
Processed Cheese					
plain	297		17.8	5	23
Cheese Slices					
singles DAIRYLEA	280		13	9.5	21
singles, light DAIRYLEA	205		17.3	8.6	10.5

Food Type	cal per 100g	cal per portion	pro (g)	carb (g)	fat (g)
Cheese Spread					
PRIMULA	226		11.7	5	17.7
WEIGHTWATCHERS	112		18.1	3.4	2.9
with roasted onion & chive					
WEIGHTWATCHERS	95		12.9	5.1	2.5
Cheese Triangles					
WEIGHTWATCHERS	117		19.9	4.3	2.2
Cheestrings					
all flavours, each (21g)					
KERRY FOODS		69	5.9	Tr	5
light, each (21g) KERRY FOODS		54	5.9	Tr	3.4
mini, each (10g) KERRY FOODS		33	2.8	Tr	2.4
Dairylea Cheese Portions					
KRAFT	240		10.5	5.3	19.5
Dairylea Cheese Strip Cheese					
KRAFT	350		21.5	1	27.5
Primula					
PRIMULA	228		12.9	2.1	18.7
cheese & chive PRIMULA	233		13	2.5	19
cheese & ham PRIMULA	232		13.5	2.1	18.8
cheese & prawn PRIMULA	220		13.3	2.7	17.3
Dairy-Free					
Benecol Dairy-Free					
each MCNEIL CONSUMER NUTRITIONAL	30	1.1	2.1	1.9	

Food Type	cal per 100g	cal per portion	pro (g)	carb (g)	fat (g)
Cream, Soya Alternative to					
ALPRO	170		2	1.6	17.2
OY					
chocolate flavour soya milkshake ALPRO	75		3.8	9.8	2.2
strawberry flavour soya milkshake ALPRO	68		3.8	8	2.2
Rice Drink					
calcium-enriched PROVAMEL	61		0.2	12.2	1.2
organic PROVAMEL	49		0.1	9.5	1.2
Soft Cheese					
plain, organic PROVAMEL	100		10	2	6
Soya Milk					
sweetened	42		3.4	2.9	1.9
unsweetened	32		3.4	0.2	1.9
banana flavour, organic PROVAMEL	195		9.5	26	5.5
chocolate flavour, organic PROVAMEL	208		9.5	28	6
fat-free SO GOOD	33		3	5	0
original, organic PROVAMEL	113		9.3	6	5.5
strawberry flavour ALPRO	62		3.3	7.9	1.8
sweetened, organic PROVAMEL	148		9.5	14.5	5.5
unsweetened, organic PROVAMEL	88		9.3	0.3	5.5

Dairy

Food Type	cal per 100g	cal per portion	pro (g)	carb (g)	fat (g)
vanilla flavoured, organic					
PROVAMEL	151		9.5	15.8	5.5
Vitalite					
DAIRY CREST	503		0	0	56
Yofu, organic					
blueberry PROVAMEL	81		3.9	10.3	2.2
cherry PROVAMEL	82		3.9	10.5	2.2
forest fruit PROVAMEL	81		3.9	10.1	2.2
peach & mango PROVAMEL	81		3.9	10.4	2.2
plain PROVAMEL	59		4.7	2.8	2.7
strawberry PROVAMEL	81		3.9	10.2	2.2

Food Type

Food Type	cal per 100g	cal per portion	pro (g)	carb (g)	fat (g)
Desserts & Puddings					
Puddings & Trifles					
Bramley Apple Crumble					
AUNT BESSIE'S	214		2.2	37.5	6.1
Bread Pudding	271		6	20.5	18.3
Christmas Pudding	329		3	56.3	11.8
Creamy Macaroni					
AMBROSIA	90		3.7	15	1.7
Jam Roly Poly					
AUNT BESSIE'S	394		6.1	55	16.6
Meringue	381		5.3	96	Tr
nests WALKERS	395		4.8	94.1	0
shells WALKERS	395		5.9	92.9	0
Pavlova					
raspberry	284		2.9	45.4	10.1
toffee	372		3.2	57.9	14.2
Profiteroles	337		5.3	31	21.3
chocolate WEIGHTWATCHERS	287		4.8	30.4	17.1
Sago Pudding					
made with semi-skimmed milk	93		4	20.1	0.2
made with whole milk	130		4.1	19.6	4.3
Semolina Pudding					
made with semi-skimmed milk	93		4	20.1	0.2
made with whole milk	130		4.1	19.6	4.3
as sold WHITWORTHS	334		11.1	69.2	1.4

Food Type	cal per 100g	cal per portion	pro (g)	carb (g)	fat (g)
Semolina Pudding Mix					
as prepared BIRD'S	142		1.9	23.9	4.3
Tapioca Pudding					
made with semi-skimmed milk	93		4	20.1	0.2
made with whole milk	130		4.1	19.6	4.3
as sold WHITWORTHS	348		0.4	86.4	0.1
Torte					
chocolate fondant GÜ	423		5.7	32	30.2
Trifle	166		2.6	21	8.1
sherry	156		2.2	19.3	8.2
chocolate CADBURY	285		5.2	24.3	18.5
Trifle Mixes					
as sold, chocolate BIRD'S	458		7.2	66.1	18.3
as sold, raspberry BIRD'S	413		2.5	76.5	10.8
as sold, strawberry BIRD'S	413		2.5	76.4	10.8
Vanilla Crème Brûlée Dessert Mix					
DR OETKER	232		2.8	25.4	13.2
Sponge & Rice Puddings					
Banoffee Desserts					
WEIGHTWATCHERS	190		4.9	34.3	3.7
Chocolate Fudge Steamed Pudding, Aunty's					
OLD FASHIONED FOODS LTD	301		3.6	58.7	4.7

Food Type	cal per 100g	cal per portion	pro (g)	carb (g)	fat (g)
Chocolate Sponge Pudding					
with Cadbury chocolate sauce,					
canned HEINZ	302		5.2	44.6	11.4
Creamed Rice					
AMBROSIA	99		3.2	16.5	2.2
caramel WEIGHTWATCHERS	87		2.7	18.1	0.4
in a pot AMBROSIA	104		3.3	17.1	2.5
low fat AMBROSIA	91		3.2	16.5	1.3
vanilla WEIGHTWATCHERS	83		3.2	16	0.7
Creamy Rice Pudding					
HEINZ	106		3.4	18.6	1.9
with sultanas & nutmeg					
AMBROSIA	107		3.3	17	2.9
traditional AMBROSIA	107		3.3	17	2.9
Creamy Semolina					
AMBROSIA	79		3.3	12.6	1.7
Creamy Tapioca					
AMBROSIA	75		2.7	12.4	1.6
Ginger Syrup Steamed					
Pudding, Aunty's					
OLD FASHIONED FOODS LTD	296		3.2	61.9	3.3
Golden Syrup Steamed					
Pudding, Aunty's					
OLD FASHIONED FOODS LTD	294		3.2	60.4	3.8

Food Type	cal per 100g	cal per portion	pro (g)	carb (g)	fat (g)
Hot Chocolate Caramel Sponge Pudding					
CADBURY	315		4	42.3	14.3
Hot Chocolate Sponge Pudding					
CADBURY	325		4	34.4	18.9
Indulgent Chocolate Sponge Pudding					
micro HEINZ	287		3.6	39	12.9
Müllerice					
MÜLLER	106		3.7	16.9	2.6
apple MÜLLER	112		3.2	19.8	2.2
blueberry MÜLLER	111		3.2	19.6	2.2
cherry MÜLLER	109		3.2	19.2	2.2
raspberry MÜLLER	109		3.2	19.1	2.2
rhubarb MÜLLER	113		3.2	20	2.2
strawberry MÜLLER	110		3.2	19.3	2.2
vanilla custard MÜLLER	115		3.4	19.8	2.5
Rice Pudding					
canned	85		3.3	16.1	1.3
organic AMBROSIA	110		3.5	15.6	3.7
with strawberry AMBROSIA	109		2.7	19.8	2
Spotted Dick					
AUNT BESSIE'S	399		6.1	49.3	19.6
Spotted Dick Sponge Pudding					
canned HEINZ	337		3.4	52.7	12.6

Food Type	cal per 100g	cal per portion	pro (g)	carb (g)	fat (g)
Spotted Dick Sponge Pudding, Delightful					
micro HEINZ	325		3.1	43.2	15.5
Sticky Toffee Pudding					
AUNT BESSIE'S	337		3.6	69.9	4.7
Sticky Toffee Steamed Pudding					
Aunty's OLD FASHIONED FOODS LTD	304		3	60.9	4.6
Strawberry Jam Sponge Pudding					
micro HEINZ	283		2	42.3	11.7
Strawberry Sponge Steamed Pudding					
Aunty's OLD FASHIONED FOODS LTD	299		3.2	60.3	4.1
Treacle Sponge Pudding					
canned HEINZ	285		2.5	50.1	8.3
super sticky, micro HEINZ	289		1.9	45.3	11.1
Chilled Desserts					
Aero Milk Chocolate Mousse					
NESTLÉ	166		4.9	22.6	6.1
Aero White Chocolate Mousse					
NESTLÉ	187		4.5	19.1	10.1
Belgian Chocolate & Vanilla Mousse					
WEIGHTWATCHERS	132		4.4	22.2	2.8

Food Type	cal per 100g	cal per portion	pro (g)	carb (g)	fat (g)
Cadbury Chocolate Mousse					
MÜLLER	195		6.1	24.6	8.2
light MÜLLER	110		4.6	14.2	3.4
Cadbury Crunchie Twinpot					
MÜLLER	260		4.4	33.4	12.2
Cadbury Flake Twinpot					
MÜLLER	240		4.4	26.6	12.6
Cadbury Trifle					
MÜLLER	285		5.2	24.3	18.5
light MÜLLER	140		4.6	20.4	4.3
Cheeky Chocolate Dessert					
_GÜ_	443		3.3	24.1	36.9
Chocolate Flavoured Soya Dessert					
ALPRO	88		3	13.6	2.3
organic, each (125g) PROVAMEL		116	3.8	20.6	0.5
Chocolate Mousse	149		4	19.9	6.5
Chocolate & Hazelnut Mousse, Creamy					
ONKEN	137		3.3	17.6	6
Crème Brûlée	324		4.3	13.9	27.9
Crème Caramel	113		3	20.6	2.1
Crunch Corner					
banana choco flakes MÜLLER	143		4.1	19.3	5.2
choco crunch MÜLLER	142		4	19.6	5

Food Type	cal per 100g	cal per portion	pro (g)	carb (g)	fat (g)
chocolate fudge cake MÜLLER	162		3.3	24.5	5.4
milk chocolate digestives MÜLLER	149		4	20.1	5.5
rhubarb crumble MÜLLER	158		3.6	22.8	5.6
strawberry crumble MÜLLER	156		3.6	22.2	5.6
strawberry orange balls MÜLLER	148		4	20.1	5.4
strawberry shortcake MÜLLER	155		3.9	21	5.8
toffee hoops MÜLLER	153		4	21.1	5.5
vanilla choco balls MÜLLER	149		4.1	20.2	5.5
Double Chocolate Brownies					
WEIGHTWATCHERS	177		5.2	32.3	3
Fruit Mousse					
creamy chocolate & hazelnut					
DR OETKER	137		3.3	17.6	6
creamy peach DR OETKER	143		5.1	15	6.7
creamy strawberry DR OETKER	143		5.1	15	6.7
fruity apple & blackberry					
DR OETKER	106		4.7	17.8	1.5
fruity lemon DR OETKER	108		4.6	17.8	1.5
Healthy Balance Corner					
red berry MÜLLER	119		5	18	2.7
strawberry MÜLLER	117		4.2	19.8	2.1
tropical MÜLLER	113		4.7	18.2	2.1
Strawberry Mousse					
ONKEN	141		5.1	14.7	6.7

Food Type	cal per 100g	cal per portion	pro (g)	carb (g)	fat (g)
Strawberry & Vanilla Mousse					
WEIGHTWATCHERS	109		3.7	18.1	2.4
Tiramisu	255		5	34	11
Ice Cream & Frozen Desserts					
Arctic Roll					
chocolate BIRDS EYE	222		3.6	38.1	6.1
raspberry BIRDS EYE	207		3	36.8	5.3
Bailey's Irish Cream Ice Cream					
HÄAGEN DAZS	226		3.7	19.3	14.7
Baked Alaska Ice Cream					
BEN & JERRY'S	260		4	29	15
Banoffee Desserts					
WEIGHTWATCHERS	190		4.9	34.3	3.7
Belgian Chocolate Cream Ice Cream					
HÄAGEN DAZS	277		3.9	23.8	18.4
Cadbury Chocolate Fudge Ice Cream Cone					
each (115ml) CADBURY		210	2.6	29	9.5
Cadbury Dairy Milk Fruit & Nut Stick					
each (90ml) CADBURY		235	2.9	23.4	14.4
Cadbury Dairy Milk Ice Cream					
CADBURY	140		2.1	18.1	6.8

Food Type	cal per 100g	cal per portion	pro (g)	carb (g)	fat (g)
Cadbury Dairy Milk Ice Cream Cones					
mint, each (115ml) CADBURY		190	2.8	24.7	8.8
Cadbury Flake 99 Ice Cream Cones					
each (125ml) CADBURY		250	3.3	30.7	12.8
Calippo					
orange, each (105ml) WALL'S		100	Tr	24	Tr
strawberry tropical, each (105ml) WALL'S		90	Tr	21	Tr
Caramel Chew Chew Ice Cream					
BEN & JERRY'S	270		3	29	16
Caramel Cinnamon Waffle Ice Cream					
CARTE D'OR	120		1.5	15	6
Caramel Crunch Desserts					
WEIGHTWATCHERS	206		4.4	35.3	5.2
Cherry Garcia Frozen Yogurt					
low fat BEN & JERRY'S	150		4	28	3
Choc Ice					
each		137	1.1	13	9
Choc Ice, Chunky					
each (75ml) WALL'S		150	2	14	10
Chocolate Brownie Sundae					
each (215g)		779	5.8	61.7	56.5

Food Type	cal per 100g	cal per portion	pro (g)	carb (g)	fat (g)
Chocolate Fudge Brownie Ice Cream					
BEN & JERRY'S	260		4	32	13
Chocolate Ice Cream					
organic GREEN & BLACK	248		5	25.3	14.1
soft scoop WALL'S	80		1.6	10	3.5
Chocolate Inspiration Ice Cream					
CARTE D'OR	120		2	15	6
Chocolate Sandwich					
each (55ml) SKINNY COW		100	1.9	16.2	3
Chocolate Top Desserts					
WEIGHTWATCHERS	221		4.7	26.5	11.5
Chunky Monkey Ice Cream					
BEN & JERRY'S	290		4	27	17
Cookie Dough Ice Cream					
BEN & JERRY'S	270		4	31	14
Cookies & Cream Ice Cream					
HÄAGEN DAZS	225		3.7	20	14.4
Cornetto					
chocolate, each (90ml) WALL'S		228	3.1	22	14
classico, each (125ml) WALL'S		250	3.5	25	15
mint, each (90ml) WALL'S		190	2.5	20	11
strawberry, each (120ml) WALL'S		200	2	29	8
Cornish Clotted Cream Ice Cream					
KELLY'S OF CORNWALL	227		3	16.2	16.2

Food Type	cal per 100g	cal per portion	pro (g)	carb (g)	fat (g)
Cream of Cornish					
WALL'S	85		1.5	10	4
Crema di Mascarpone Ice Cream					
CARTE D'OR	207		2.8	29	8.9
Double Chocolate Brownies					
WEIGHTWATCHERS	177		5.2	32.3	3
Dulce de Leche Ice Cream					
HÄAGEN DAZS	239		3.9	24.1	14.1
Fab					
each (58ml) NESTLÉ		79	0.3	13.2	2.7
Feast					
chocolate, each (92ml) WALL'S		280	3	20	20
mint, each (92ml) WALL'S		280	3	20	20
Fruit Pastilles Ice Lolly					
each (65ml) NESTLÉ		60	0.1	14.9	Tr
Golden Syrup Ice Cream					
TATE & LYLE	140		2.4	17.8	6.6
Greek Yoghurt & Honey Ice Cream					
CARTE D'OR	120		1.5	16	5
Half Baked Ice Cream					
BEN & JERRY'S	270		5	26	13
Honeycomb Chunks Dairy Ice Cream					
KELLY'S OF CORNWALL	238		3.7	27	12.8

Food Type	cal per 100g	cal per portion	pro (g)	carb (g)	fat (g)
Ice Cream Stick					
chocolate coated, each (90ml)					
LYONS MAID		214	2.8	18.9	14.1
Ice Smoothie					
mango, each (90ml) DEL MONTE		97	0.1	23.8	0.1
raspberry, each (90ml) DEL MONTE		96	0.1	23.8	0.1
Lavazza Latte Macchiato					
Ice Cream					
CARTE D'OR	120		1.5	16	5
Magnum					
almond, each (120ml) WALL'S		280	4.5	26	18
classic, each (120ml) WALL'S		260	3.5	25	16
double caramel, each (120ml)					
WALL'S		340	3.5	36	20
mint, each (110ml) WALL'S		260	3.5	26	16
white, each (120ml) WALL'S		260	3.5	26	16
Magnum Mini					
almond, each (60ml) WALL'S		180	2.5	16	11
chocolate, each (60ml) WALL'S		170	2	14	11
classic, each (60ml) WALL'S		170	2	15	11
strawberry, each (60ml) WALL'S		170	2	14	11
white, each (60ml) WALL'S		170	2.5	17	10
Magnum Origins					
Ecuador Dark, each (330ml) WALL'S		264	3.5	23	17

Food Type	cal per 100g	cal per portion	pro (g)	carb (g)	fat (g)
Mayan Mystica, each (330ml)					
WALL'S		282	3.5	26	18
Magnum Temptation					
caramel & almonds, each					
(80ml) WALL'S		240	3	24	14
chocolate, each (80ml) WALL'S		240	3	24	14
Maltesers Ice Cream					
each (45ml) MARS		113	1.3	11.3	7
Mango Smoothie Ice Cream					
DEL MONTE	107		0.2	26.5	0.1
Mars Ice Cream Bar					
each (51ml) MARS		143	1.8	15.4	8.3
Mars 'Xtra Ice Cream Bar					
each (80ml) MARS		226	2.9	24.5	13
Mascarpone Ice Cream					
CARTE D'OR	207		2.7	29	8.9
Mint Choc Chip Ice Cream					
soft scoop WALL'S	88		1.4	12	3.9
Mint Double Chocolate Sticks					
each (110ml) SKINNY COW		94	3	16.6	14.9
Mivvi					
each (90ml) NESTLÉ		92	1.2	14.2	3.4
Neapolitan Ice Cream					
soft scoop WALL'S	77		1.4	10	3.4

Food Type	cal per 100g	cal per portion	pro (g)	carb (g)	fat (g)
Phish Food Ice Cream					
BEN & JERRY'S	260		3.5	36	13
Pralines & Cream Ice Cream					
HÄAGEN DAZS	245		3.6	25.2	14.5
Raspberry Ripple Ice Cream					
soft scoop WALL'S	86		1.3	12	3.5
Raspberry Smoothie Ice Cream					
DEL MONTE	107		0.1	26.5	0.1
Snickers Ice Cream Bar					
each (63ml) MARS		220	4.5	20.4	13.4
Snickers 'Xtra Ice Cream Bar					
each (79.5ml) MARS		277	5.6	25.8	16.9
Solero					
Berry Berry, each (90ml) WALL'S		100	0.6	20	1
Exotic, each (90ml) WALL'S		99	1.3	18	2.3
Strawberry & Banana Smoothie, each (90ml) WALL'S		99	1.5	19	2.5
Sorbet					
fruit	97		0.2	24.8	0.3
lemon	128		0	32	0
Blackcurrant CARTE D'OR	78		0.4	19	0
Elderflower BOTTLEGREEN	118		0.2	29	0.1
Lemon CARTE D'OR	78		0.3	19	0
Mango CARTE D'OR	75		0.3	18	0.1

Food Type	cal per 100g	cal per portion	pro (g)	carb (g)	fat (g)
Mango Berry Swirl BEN & JERRY'S	100		0.2	25	0
Strawberry Cheesecake Frozen Yogurt					
low-fat BEN & JERRY'S	170		4	31	3
Strawberry Cheesecake Ice Cream					
BEN & JERRY'S	240		4	29	12
HÄAGEN DAZS	236		3.3	25.1	13.6
Strawberry Frozen Yogurt					
organic YEO VALLEY	140		4.8	23.5	3
Strawberry & Yoghurt Délice Ice Cream					
CARTE D'OR	95		0.9	18	2.5
Summer Berries & Cream Ice Cream					
HÄAGEN DAZS	228		2.5	24.4	13.3
Tiramisu Ice Cream					
HÄAGEN DAZS	255		3.8	23.5	16.3
Toffee Crisp Ice Cream Bar					
each (60ml) NESTLÉ		165	1.9	16.5	10.1
Toffee Flavour & Toffee Sauce Iced Dessert					
WEIGHTWATCHERS	163		2.7	26.2	4.8
Toffee & Honeycomb Sundaes					
each (330ml) WEIGHTWATCHERS		122	1.7	27	2.6

Food Type	cal per 100g	cal per portion	pro (g)	carb (g)	fat (g)
Triple Chocolate Ice Cream Sticks					
each (110ml) SKINNY COW		87	2.9	15.4	1.5
Twix 'Extra' Ice Cream					
per finger (42.5g) MARS		208	2	27.8	10.1
Vanilla Caramel Nut Ice Cream					
organic GREEN & BLACK	250		4.1	26.5	14.2
Vanilla Ice Cream					
CARTE D'OR	100		1.5	14	4.5
HÄAGEN DAZS	225		3.8	18.1	15.2
MACKIES	193		4	18	11
Cornish KELLY'S OF CORNWALL	223		5	21	13
diabetic FRANK'S	163		3.4	17.9	7.7
Fairtrade BEN & JERRY'S	230		4	20	15
light CARTE D'OR	68		1.2	11	2.2
organic GREEN & BLACK	219		4.5	20.2	13.3
organic YEO VALLEY	209		5.1	21.8	11.3
soft scoop WALL'S	85		1.3	10.4	4
soft scoop, light WALL'S	62		1.3	7	2.6
with chocolate sauce, organic GREEN & BLACK	240		4.3	24.6	13.9
Viennetta					
mint WALL'S	133		1.8	12	8.6
vanilla WALL'S	120		1.5	12	8

Food Type	cal per 100g	cal per portion	pro (g)	carb (g)	fat (g)
White Chocolate & Raspberry Swirl Ice Cream					
organic GREEN & BLACK	210		4.1	19.5	12.8
Cheesecake					
Banoffee Cheesecake	310		5.4	36.5	15.4
Berry & Vanilla Cheesecake					
FRÜ	286		3.3	27.8	17.8
Blackcurrant Cheesecake					
CREAMFIELDS	276		5.2	32.8	13.8
DEVONSHIRE	278		4	34.3	13.9
Blueberry Cheesecake					
FRÜ	285		3	28.5	17.5
Chocolate Cheesecake	376		5.7	39.9	21.5
Chocolate & Vanilla Cheesecake					
GÜ	483		3.3	28.9	34
Lemon Cheesecake	354		4.3	31.2	23.5
FRÜ	373		3.8	32.1	26.1
Mandarin Cheesecake					
Low-Fat	189		4	32	5
New York Vanilla Cheesecake	345		6.4	28.2	22.7
Raspberry Cheesecake	299		3.8	39.1	15.4
Sticky Toffee Cheesecake	375		4	35.3	24.2
Strawberry Cheesecake					
HEINZ	268		4.3	31.7	13.8

Food Type	cal per 100g	cal per portion	pro (g)	carb (g)	fat (g)
Strawberry Cheesecake					
WEIGHTWATCHERS	179		5	32.6	3.2
Strawberries & Cream Cheesecake					
DEVONSHIRE	279		3.9	31.4	15.3
Summer Fruits Cheesecake					
low fat	186		3.5	33	4.4
Toffee Apple Cheesecake	301		5.4	34.4	15.8
Jelly					
Jelly					
all varieties, made with					
water	61		1.2	15.1	0
all varieties, as sold HARTLEY'S	296		4.2	69.8	0
Jelly Pots Ready To Eat					
all flavours, each (125g)					
HARTLEY'S		8	0	2	0
all flavours, low sugar, each					
(175g) HARTLEY'S		5	0	1	0.1
Orange & Peach Flavour Jelly Crystals					
as sold WEIGHTWATCHERS	7		Tr	1.4	0.1
Strawberry & Raspberry Flavour Jelly Crystals					
as sold WEIGHTWATCHERS	7		Tr	1.4	0.1

Food Type	cal per 100g	cal per portion	pro (g)	carb (g)	fat (g)
Dessert Powders					
Instant Dessert Powder					
as sold	391		2.4	60.1	17.3
made up with whole milk		111	3.1	14.8	6.3
Angel Delight					
banana, as sold BIRD'S	490		2.5	72	21
butterscotch, as sold BIRD'S	469		2.1	73.4	18.5
butterscotch, no added sugar, as sold BIRD'S	474		4.2	61.6	23.5
chocolate, as sold BIRD'S	464		3.4	73	17.6
raspberry, as sold BIRD'S	483		2.4	71.2	20.9
strawberry, as sold BIRD'S	482		2.4	71.5	20.7
strawberry, no added sugar, as sold BIRD'S	487		4.6	58.9	25.9
Blancmange Powder					
chocolate, as sold PEARCE DUFF	100		2.9	14.4	3.6
raspberry, as sold PEARCE DUFF	100		2.9	14.4	3.6
strawberry, as sold PEARCE DUFF	100		2.9	14.4	3.6
vanilla, as sold PEARCE DUFF	100		2.9	14.4	3.6
Custard Desserts					
Ambrosia Layers					
caramel AMBROSIA	114		2.5	19.6	2.9
chocolate AMBROSIA	118		2.8	20.2	2.8
rhubarb compote AMBROSIA	96		2.5	16.7	2.2

Desserts & Puddings

Food Type	cal per 100g	cal per portion	pro (g)	carb (g)	fat (g)
Caramel Flavoured Soya Dessert					
organic, each (125g) PROVAMEL		124	3.8	22.3	2.1
Custard Dessert Pot					
chocolate flavour AMBROSIA	114		3.2	18.5	3
strawberry flavour AMBROSIA	103		2.8	16.7	2.8
vanilla flavour AMBROSIA	102		2.8	16.4	2.8
Dark Chocolate Flavoured Soya Dessert					
ALPRO	92		3	14.6	2.2
Devon Custard Dessert Pot					
low-fat AMBROSIA	70		3.1	11.9	1.1
ready to eat AMBROSIA	102		2.9	16	2.9
Mocha Flavoured Soya Dessert					
organic, each (125g) PROVAMEL		118	3.8	20.4	2.3
Vanilla Flavoured Soya Dessert					
ALPRO	80		3	12.7	1.8
organic, each (125g) PROVAMEL		114	3.8	19.5	2.3
Sweet Sauces & Toppings					
Belgian Chocolate Sauce					
ENGLISH PROVENDER CO.	370		2.2	49.3	18.2
Brandy Flavour Sauce Mix					
as sold BIRD'S	423		6.1	78.4	9.4
Chocolate Flavoured Custard					
in pots AMBROSIA	114		3.2	18.5	3

Food Type	cal per 100g	cal per portion	pro (g)	carb (g)	fat (g)
Custard					
canned	100		3	14	4
made up with skimmed milk		79	3.8	16.8	0.1
made up with whole milk		118	3.9	16.2	4.5
ready to serve	101		2.8	16	2.9
ready to serve AUNT BESSIE'S	105		2.9	15.6	3.4
ready to serve HEINZ	100		2.5	15.7	3
Custard Powder					
as sold BIRD'S	339		0.4	84.2	Tr
Custard, Chocolate					
organic, per serving (175g)					
PROVAMEL		166	5.3	29.2	3
Custard, Dairy-Free					
ready to serve ALPRO	81		3	13	1.8
Custard, Instant					
as sold BIRD'S	425		4.3	76.3	11.4
low-fat, as sold BIRD'S	407		4.3	79	8.2
Custard, Vanilla					
organic, per serving (175g)					
PROVAMEL		161	5.3	27.7	3.2
Devon Custard					
canned or carton AMBROSIA	102		2.9	16	2.9
low-fat, canned or carton					
AMBROSIA	70		3.1	11.9	1.1

Food Type	cal per 100g	cal per portion	pro (g)	carb (g)	fat (g)
Dream Topping					
made up BIRD'S	356		1.8	4.7	6.6
made up, sugar-free BIRD'S	85		1.8	4.3	6.3
Dulce de Leche Chocolate Toffee Sauce					
MERCHANT GOURMET	297		3.8	57.7	5.7
Maple Syrup					
organic MERIDIAN FOODS LTD	334		Tr	85.3	Tr
Raspberry Coulis					
ENGLISH PROVENDER CO.	110		0.9	26.5	0.1
Rum Flavour Sauce					
ready to eat BIRD'S	91		2.9	16.1	1.4
Tip Top					
NESTLÉ	107		3.5	8.6	6.4
squirty NESTLÉ	276		2.4	8	26
Treat					
crackin' ASKEY'S	622		3.3	47	4.8
maple ASKEY'S	308		Tr	77	0.1
milk chocolate ASKEY'S	375		1.1	66.8	11.5
strawberry ASKEY'S	309		Tr	77	0.1
toffee ASKEY'S	323		1.6	76	0.1

Food Type	cal per 100g	cal per portion	pro (g)	carb (g)	fat (g)
Dips & Pre-dressed Salads					
BBQ Dipping Sauce					
BLUE DRAGON	76		1	17.9	0
Beetroot Salad	65		0.7	12.8	0.8
Bengal Spiced Tomato & Red Pepper Dip					
SHARWOOD	114		0.8	26.9	0.3
Chilli & Mango Dipping Sauce					
BLUE DRAGON	215		0.5	54	0.1
Chilli & Pineapple Dipping Sauce					
BLUE DRAGON	213		0.5	54	0.1
Coleslaw					
creamy	181		0.9	6	17
reduced fat	89		1.7	7	6
with cheese	242		4.8	6.3	22
Coronation Chicken	229		11	8	17
Couscous Salad					
spicy	130		3.6	25.1	1.7
with roast vegetables	149		4.4	21.7	4.9
Dairylea Dunkers					
Baked Crisps KRAFT	225		9.2	26	8.9
Breadstick KRAFT	235		10.5	28	8.6
Jumbo Tubes KRAFT	255		9.2	26	12.5
Nachos KRAFT	255		9	22.5	14
Salt & Vinegar Twists KRAFT	215		8.9	18.5	11.5

Food Type	cal per 100g	cal per portion	pro (g)	carb (g)	fat (g)
Dipping Relish					
crushed tomato BAXTERS	144		1.5	31	1.5
cucumber & mint BAXTERS	139		0.5	34	0.1
red pepper & pineapple BAXTERS	147		0.8	35.2	0.3
spicy red onion BAXTERS	117		0.9	27.4	0.4
Fiery Guava Dipping Sauce					
LEVI ROOTS	128		0.4	31.5	Tr
Florida Salad	180		0.8	8.2	15.6
Green Label Mango Chutney & Chilli Dip					
SHARWOOD	233		0.3	57.8	Tr
Guacamole Dip					
DISCOVERY FOODS	140		1.2	8.6	12.2
OLD EL PASO	87		2.3	8.5	4.8
Houmous	369		7	11	33
YARDEN	335		6.5	12	29
Malaysian Satay Dipping Sauce					
BLUE DRAGON	158		5.6	14.5	8.6
Nacho Cheese Dip					
PRIMULA	248		3.3	4.9	23.9
Nachos Cheese Sauce					
hot DISCOVERY FOODS	182		4.2	7.9	14.8
Nuoc Cham Nem Dipping Sauce					
BLUE DRAGON	151		1.5	36.2	0.1

Food Type	cal per 100g	cal per portion	pro (g)	carb (g)	fat (g)
Pasta Salad					
cheese pasta salad	259		5.1	15.3	19.7
chicken & bacon Caesar pasta					
salad	256		8.3	14.1	18.5
Italian pasta salad	140		3.5	22.6	3.7
prawn pasta salad	195		4.9	18.9	11.1
tuna & sweetcorn pasta salad	205		7.2	20.5	10
Peanut Satay Dipping Sauce					
AMOY	208		5	18.4	12.7
Potato Salad	165		1.3	9.5	13.5
Roasted Garlic Dip					
PRIMULA	243		3	3.8	24
Salsa					
Hot DISCOVERY FOODS	56		1.3	11.7	0.4
Hot DORITOS	40		0.9	8.5	0.2
Hot, Original OLD EL PASO	43		1.6	9.1	0.5
Hot, Taco OLD EL PASO	40		2.4	7	0.2
Medium DISCOVERY FOODS	56		1.4	11.7	0.4
Mild DORITOS	40		0.9	8.5	0.2
Mild, Original OLD EL PASO	43		1.6	9.1	0.5
Roasted Tomato & Pepper					
OLD EL PASO	37		1.3	8	0.5
Tequila & Lime DISCOVERY FOODS	36		1.5	10.2	0.2
Sour Cream Based Dips	360		2.9	4	37

Food Type	cal per 100g	cal per portion	pro (g)	carb (g)	fat (g)
Sour Cream & Chive Dip					
DORITOS	260		1.9	7	25
PRIMULA	238		2.9	3.6	23.6
Spicy Salsa Dip					
PRIMULA	152		0.6	8.1	0.1
Splendips					
Chive Crackers & Tomato Chutney Philadelphia KRAFT	180		7.9	27	4
Nachos & Tomato Salsa Philadelphia KRAFT	175		6.3	20	7.5
Poppadoms & Mango Chutney Philadelphia KRAFT	171		5.1	26.5	4.7
Rice Crackers & Sweet Chilli Dip Philadelphia KRAFT	194		6.1	37	2.2
Spring Onion Dip					
PRIMULA	236		3	5.1	22.6
Sweet Chilli Dipping Sauce					
BLUE DRAGON	229		0.6	55.1	0.7
hot BLUE DRAGON	229		0.6	55.1	0.7
with kaffir lime BLUE DRAGON	229		0.6	55.1	0.2
Sweet Red Chilli Dip					
SHARWOOD	104		0.7	24.8	0.2
Sweet Soy & Sesame Dipping Sauce					
AMOY	146		0.7	32.8	1.3

Food Type	cal per 100g	cal per portion	pro (g)	carb (g)	fat (g)
Sweet & Sour Dipping Sauce					
AMOY	96		0.4	22.9	0.1
BLUE DRAGON	105		0.3	25.4	0
Taramasalata Dip	262		1.3	3.5	27
Thai Sweet Chilli Dipping Sauce					
AMOY	142		0.5	34.2	0.2
SHARWOOD	137		0.3	31.4	1.1
Three Bean Salad	104		7.1	13.6	2.3
Tzatziki	132		5.1	4.9	10.2
FAGE	92		3.2	4.1	7

Food Type	cal per 100g/ml	cal per portion	pro (g)	carb (g)	fat (g)
Drinks (Alcoholic)					
Advocaat	272		4.7	28.4	6.3
Bols	257		3.4	27	5.6
Bailey's Irish Cream					
50ml		175	n/a	n/a	n/a
Beer, bitter					
best/premium	33		0.3	2.2	Tr
canned	32		0.3	2.3	Tr
draught	32		0.3	2.3	Tr
keg	31		0.3	2.3	Tr
Beer, mild					
draught	25		0.2	1.6	Tr
Beer					
John Smith's 500ml		175	n/a	n/a	n/a
Lowenbräu 340ml		160	n/a	n/a	n/a
Old Speckled Hen 500ml		225	n/a	n/a	n/a
Tetley's Bitter 440ml		167	n/a	n/a	n/a
Brandy	222		Tr	Tr	0
Breezer, Bacardi					
all flavours 275ml bottle		198	n/a	n/a	n/a
Brown Ale					
Newcastle 500ml		200	n/a	n/a	n/a
Cherry Brandy	255		Tr	32.6	0
Cider					
dry	36		Tr	2.6	0

Food Type	cal per 100g/ml	cal per portion	pro (g)	carb (g)	fat (g)
sweet	42		Tr	4.3	0
vintage	101		Tr	7.3	0
Scrumpy Jack HP BULMER		225	n/a	2.64	n/a
Strongbow HP BULMER		215	n/a	1.47	n/a
Woodpecker HP BULMER		210	n/a	2.38	n/a
Cognac					
Courvoisier 50ml		111	n/a	n/a	n/a
Cointreau					
50ml		170	n/a	n/a	n/a
Curaçao	311		Tr	28.3	0
Drambuie					
50ml		136	n/a	n/a	n/a
Gin	222		Tr	Tr	0
Gordon's 50ml		104	n/a	n/a	n/a
Grand Marnier	320		n/a	n/a	n/a
Lager					
bottled	29		0.2	1.5	Tr
Beck's 330ml bottle		142	n/a	n/a	n/a
Carlsberg 440ml bottle		150	n/a	n/a	n/a
Carlsberg Export 440ml bottle		189	n/a	n/a	n/a
Heineken 440ml bottle		189	n/a	n/a	n/a
Miller's Genuine Draft 340ml bottle		143	n/a	n/a	n/a
Tennent's 500ml		145	n/a	n/a	n/a

Food Type	cal per 100g/ml	cal per portion	pro (g)	carb (g)	fat (g)
Pale Ale					
bottled	28		0.3	2	Tr
Port	157		0.1	12	0
Cockburn Special Reserve 50ml		76	n/a	n/a	n/a
Rum	222		Tr	Tr	0
Bacardi, white 50ml		104	n/a	n/a	n/a
Captain Morgan, dark 50ml		111	n/a	n/a	n/a
Shandy					
canned BASS	22		Tr	4.6	0
Shandy, Bitter					
canned BEN SHAW'S	22		Tr	5.5	Tr
Sherry					
dry	116		0.2	1.4	0
medium	116		0.1	5.9	0
sweet	136		0.3	6.9	0
Harvey's Bristol Cream 50ml		77	n/a	n/a	n/a
Southern Comfort					
50ml		104	n/a	n/a	n/a
Stout					
bottled	37		0.3	4.2	Tr
extra	39		0.3	2.1	Tr
Guinness draught 500 ml		185	n/a	n/a	n/a
Strong Ale	72		0.7	6.1	Tr
Tequila					
Jose Cuervo 50ml		105	n/a	n/a	n/a

Food Type	cal per 100g/ml	cal per portion	pro (g)	carb (g)	fat (g)
Tia Lusso					
50ml		126	n/a	n/a	n/a
Tia Maria					
50ml		131	n/a	n/a	n/a
Vermouth					
Martini Bianco 50ml		73	n/a	n/a	n/a
Martini Extra Dry 50ml		48	n/a	n/a	n/a
Martini Rosso 50ml		70	n/a	n/a	n/a
Vintage Cider: see CIDER					
Vodka	222		Tr	Tr	0
Smirnoff Ice 275ml bottle		187	n/a	n/a	n/a
Smirnoff Red 50ml		104	n/a	n/a	n/a
Whiskey					
Jack Daniel's, blended 50ml		111	n/a	n/a	n/a
Whisky	222		Tr	Tr	0
Laphroaig, single malt	222		n/a	n/a	n/a
Teacher's, blended 50ml		111	n/a	n/a	n/a
Wine					
red	68		0.1	0.2	0
rosé	71		0.1	2.5	0
white, dry	66		0.1	0.6	0
white, medium	74		0.1	3	0
white, sparkling	74		0.3	5.1	0
white, sweet	94		0.2	5.9	0

Food Type	cal per 100g/ml	cal per portion	pro (g)	carb (g)	fat (g)
Wine, sparkling					
Asti Spumante 125ml		95	n/a	n/a	n/a
Champagne					
Bollinger 125ml		95	n/a	n/a	n/a
Wine					
white, Chardonnay 125ml					
WOLF BLASS		93	n/a	n/a	n/a
white, Pinot Grigio 125ml					
TRULLI		93	n/a	n/a	n/a
WKD					
all flavours, 275ml bottle		264	n/a	n/a	n/a

Food Type	cal per 100g	cal per portion	pro (g)	carb (g)	fat (g)
Drinks (Non-alcoholic)					
Juices & Cordials					
Apple Juice					
unsweetened	38		0.1	9.9	0.1
DEL MONTE	47		0.3	10.8	Tr
cloudy COPELLA	47		0	11.7	0
concentrate, organic MERIDIAN					
FOODS	383		0.5	92.4	0.6
English CAWSTON VALE	44		0.4	10.3	0.1
organic LIBBY	47		0.1	11.2	Tr
pressed BRITVIC	49		0.1	11	0.1
Apple Juice Drink					
High Juice ROBINSONS	210		0.1	51	Tr
Apple, Blueberry & Aronia					
Juice Concentrate					
organic MERIDIAN FOODS	381		1.8	92	0.8
Apple, Cherry & Raspberry Drink					
High Juice ROBINSONS	196		0.2	48	0.1
Apple, Cranberry & Aronia					
Juice Concentrate					
organic MERIDIAN FOODS	357		0.5	88	0.4
Apple, Strawberry & Lychee,					
undiluted					
High Juice ROBINSONS	194		0.1	48	0.1

Food Type	cal per 100g/ml	cal per portion	pro (g)	carb (g)	fat (g)
Apple & Blackcurrant Drink					
ROBINSONS	43		0.1	9.8	Tr
no added sugar ROBINSONS	9		0.1	1.2	Tr
Apple & Blackcurrant Juice					
CAWSTON VALE	44		0.5	10	0.1
COPELLA	53		0	12.8	0
concentrate, MERIDIAN FOODS	229		0.5	57.4	Tr
Fruit Shoot 100% ROBINSONS	44		0.2	10.2	0.1
J20	45		0.1	10.6	0.1
Apple & Cranberry Fruit Spring					
BRITVIC	6		Tr	1	Tr
Apple & Cranberry Fruit Spring Drink					
ROBINSONS	39.1		Tr	9.3	Tr
Apple & Elderflower Juice					
CAWSTON VALE	43		0.4	10.2	0.1
COPELLA	45		0	11.2	0
Apple & Ginger Juice					
CAWSTON VALE	44		0.4	10.3	0.1
Apple & Mango Juice					
COPELLA	46		0	11.6	0
Apple & Mango Juice Drink					
J20	43		0.1	10	0.1
Apple & Melon Juice Drink					
J20	39		0.1	9.2	0.1

Food Type	cal per 100g/ml	cal per portion	pro (g)	carb (g)	fat (g)
Apple & Pear Juice					
COPELLA	44		0	10.7	0
Apple & Raspberry Juice					
COPELLA	44		0.7	10.2	0
Apple & Raspberry Juice Drink					
J2O	49		0.1	11.4	0.1
Apple & Rhubarb Juice					
CAWSTON VALE	46		0.2	9.7	0.4
Barley Water					
lemon, original ROBINSONS	96		0.3	21.8	Tr
orange, original ROBINSONS	98		0.3	23.1	0.1
Blackberry & Russet Apple Cordial					
diluted (100ml) BOTTLEGREEN		22	0	5.6	Tr
Blackcurrant Cordial					
BRITVIC	63		Tr	14.7	0
Blackcurrant Juice Drink					
diluted (100ml) RIBENA		46	n/a	11.4	n/a
ready to drink, each (288ml)					
RIBENA		147	Tr	36.3	0
really light, ready to drink, each (200ml) RIBENA		8	0.1	1	0
Blackcurrant Squash					
undiluted, organic ROCK'S	240		0.1	61	Tr

Food Type	cal per 100g/ml	cal per portion	pro (g)	carb (g)	fat (g)
Blackcurrant & Raspberry Fruit Spring					
BRITVIC	4		0.1	0.7	Tr
Blueberry Juice Drink					
really light RIBENA	3		n/a	0.5	n/a
Blood Orange Drink					
High Juice, undiluted ROBINSONS	217		0.3	52	Tr
Blood Orange & Mandarin Cordial					
organic BELVOIR	186		0.3	46.1	0.1
Capri-Sun 100% Juice					
apple CAPRI-SUN	39.7		0	10.3	0.1
orange CAPRI-SUN	37.6		0	9.2	0.1
summer fruits CAPRI-SUN	51.7		0.2	11.6	0
Capri-Sun Juice Drink					
apple CAPRI-SUN	46		0	11.1	0
blackcurrant CAPRI-SUN	53		0	12.8	0
orange CAPRI-SUN	43.2		0	10.5	0
summer berries CAPRI-SUN	44		0	10.6	0
tropical CAPRI-SUN	44		0	10.6	0
Carrot Juice	24		0.5	5.7	0.1
Cox's Apple & Plum Cordial					
diluted (100ml) BOTTLEGREEN		22	0	5.6	Tr
Cranberry Cordial					
undiluted, organic ROCK'S	251		0.1	63	Tr

Food Type	cal per 100g/ml	cal per portion	pro (g)	carb (g)	fat (g)
Cranberry Juice					
classic OCEAN SPRAY	49		0	11.6	Tr
Cranberry Juice					
light	8		0	1.4	0
Cranberry for Water					
classic OCEAN SPRAY	92		0.1	22.1	Tr
light OCEAN SPRAY	32		0.1	7.1	Tr
Cranberry & Blackcurrant Juice Drink					
OCEAN SPRAY	52		Tr	12.6	Tr
Cranberry & Blueberry Juice Drink					
OCEAN SPRAY	48		Tr	11.5	Tr
Cranberry & Mango Juice Drink					
light OCEAN SPRAY	9		0	2	0
Cranberry & Pomegranate for Water					
OCEAN SPRAY	95		Tr	23	Tr
Cranberry & Pomegranate Juice Drink					
OCEAN SPRAY	48		Tr	11.5	Tr
Cranberry & Raspberry for Water					
OCEAN SPRAY	93		0.2	22.5	Tr

Food Type	cal per 100g/ml	cal per portion	pro (g)	carb (g)	fat (g)
Cranberry & Raspberry Juice Drink					
OCEAN SPRAY	52		Tr	12.6	Tr
Dandelion & Burdock Cordial					
undiluted, organic ROCK'S	292		1.8	69	0.5
Elderflower Cordial					
diluted BOTTLEGREEN		22	0	5.6	Tr
undiluted, organic ROCK'S	345		0.3	68	0.2
Five Alive					
berry blast COCA-COLA	53		0	13	0
citrus burst COCA-COLA	34		Tr	8	0
tropical hit COCA-COLA	37		0	9	0
Fruit Punch Cordial					
undiluted, organic ROCK'S	261		0.2	65	0.3
Fruit Shoot					
apple, each (200ml) ROBINSONS		94	Tr	22.6	Tr
apple, no added sugar, each (200ml) ROBINSONS		12	Tr	2.2	Tr
blackcurrant & apple, each (200ml) ROBINSONS		92	0.2	22	Tr
blackcurrant & apple, no added sugar, each (200ml) ROBINSONS		10	0.2	1.6	Tr
orange, each (200ml) ROBINSONS		96	0.1	24	Tr

Food Type	cal per 100g/ml	cal per portion	pro (g)	carb (g)	fat (g)
orange, no added sugar, each (200ml) ROBINSONS		12	0.2	2	Tr
orange & peach, each (200ml) ROBINSONS		86	0.2	20.4	Tr
orange & peach, no added sugar, each (200ml) ROBINSONS		10	0.2	1.6	Tr
strawberry, each (200ml) ROBINSONS		90	0.2	21.2	0
strawberry, no added sugar, each (200ml) ROBINSONS		10	0.2	1.2	0
summer fruits, no added sugar, each (200ml)		10	0.2	1.2	Tr
tropical, no added sugar, each (200ml)		12	0.2	2	Tr
Fruit Shoot H2O					
apple, each (300ml) ROBINSONS		3	0	0	0
blackcurrant, each (300ml) ROBINSONS		6	0	0	0
orange, each (300ml) ROBINSONS		3	0	0	0
Fruit & Barley					
orange ROBINSONS	12		0.2	1.7	Tr
peach ROBINSONS	12		0.3	1.7	Tr
pink grapefruit ROBINSONS	15		0.3	2	Tr
strawberry & kiwi ROBINSONS	15		0.2	1.4	Tr
summer fruits ROBINSONS	14		0.2	2.1	0

Food Type	cal per 100g/ml	cal per portion	pro (g)	carb (g)	fat (g)
Ginger Cordial					
undiluted, organic ROCK'S	298		0.1	74	0.1
Ginger & Lemongrass Cordial					
diluted (100ml) BOTTLEGREEN		22	0	5.6	Tr
Grape Juice					
unsweetened	46		0.3	11.7	0.1
Grape & Melon Juice					
undiluted, High Juice ROBINSONS	187		0.2	52	0.1
Grapefruit Juice					
unsweetened	33		0.4	8.3	0.1
BRITVIC	40		0.5	8.2	0.1
Grapefruit Juice, Golden					
TROPICANA	37		0.6	7.5	0
Lemon Cordial					
undiluted, organic ROCK'S	234		0.2	58	Tr
Lemon Squash					
no sugar added ROBINSONS	10		0.2	0.3	Tr
undiluted, organic ROCK'S	192		0.1	48	Tr
Lime Cordial					
BRITVIC	46		0.1	9.1	Tr
undiluted, organic ROCK'S	234		0.2	58	Tr
Lime Cordial, Sweet					
diluted (100ml) BOTTLEGREEN		26	0	6.2	Tr
Lime Juice Cordial					
undiluted	112		0.1	29.8	0

Food Type	cal per 100g/ml	cal per portion	pro (g)	carb (g)	fat (g)
ROSE'S	21		0	4.9	0
Mango & Papaya World Fruits Juice Drink					
DEL MONTE	58		0.2	14.1	Tr
Oasis					
citrus punch COCA-COLA	28		0	6.7	0
summer fruits COCA-COLA	25		0	6	0
summer fruits, light COCA-COLA	5		n/a	0.9	n/a
Orange 'C'					
LIBBY	43		0.1	10.2	Tr
Orange Cordial					
BRITVIC	63		0.2	13.9	Tr
Orange Drink					
undiluted	107		Tr	28.5	0
Orange Fruit Squash					
undiluted ROBINSONS	54		0.2	12.2	Tr
Orange Fruit Squash					
undiluted, no added sugar					
ROBINSONS	8		0.2	0.6	Tr
Orange Juice					
unsweetened	36		0.5	8.8	0.1
BRITVIC	45		0.5	9.8	0.1
DEL MONTE	44		0.6	9.9	Tr
Fruit Shoot 100% ROBINSONS	46		0.5	9.9	0.1
no bits TROPICANA	43		0.7	9	0

Food Type	cal per 100g/ml	cal per portion	pro (g)	carb (g)	fat (g)
squeezed BRITVIC	45		190	0.5	0.1
with juicy bits TROPICANA	43		0.7	9	0
Orange Juice, Essentials					
with calcium TROPICANA	43		0.7	9	0
Orange Squash					
undiluted, High Juice ROBINSONS	182		0.3	44	Tr
undiluted, organic ROCK'S	197		0.2	49	Tr
Orange, Grape & Cranberry					
TROPICANA	46		0.4	10.4	Tr
Orange & Mandarin Fruit Spring					
BRITVIC	6		0.1	0.8	Tr
Orange & Mango Juice					
TROPICANA	45		0.8	9.6	0.1
Orange & Passionfruit Juice Drink					
J20	44		0.5	9.7	0.1
Orange & Pineapple Fruit Squash					
ROBINSONS	53		0.1	11.8	Tr
no added sugar ROBINSONS	8		0.2	0.7	Tr
Peach Drink					
undiluted, High Juice ROBINSONS	181		0.6	43.4	0.1
Pear Juice Concentrate					
MERIDIAN FOODS	272		0.4	67.3	0.1
Pear & Elderflower Cordial, Williams					
diluted (100ml) BOTTLEGREEN		22	0	5.6	Tr

Food Type	cal per 100g/ml	cal per portion	pro (g)	carb (g)	fat (g)
Pineapple Juice					
unsweetened	41		0.3	10.5	0.1
BRITVIC	50		0.3	11	0.1
Gold DEL MONTE	51		0.3	12.1	Tr
Pineapple & Guava Juice					
TROPICANA	53		0.3	12.3	0
Pink Grapefruit Drink					
undiluted, High Juice ROBINSONS	189		0.2	45	0.1
Pink Grapefruit Juice					
TROPICANA	40		0.6	8	0
Pomegranate, Grape & Apple					
TROPICANA	44		3	10.3	0
Pomegranate & Elderflower Cordial					
diluted (100ml) BOTTLEGREEN		22	0	5.6	Tr
Raspberry & Blackberry Blend					
RIBENA	53		Tr	12.7	0.1
Raspberry & Pomegranate Squash					
really light, diluted (100ml) RIBENA		3	n/a	0.5	n/a
Red Five Super Fruits Squash					
undiluted, organic ROCK'S	259		0.1	64	Tr
Ruby Breakfast					
TROPICANA	43		0.7	9	0

Food Type	cal per 100g/ml	cal per portion	pro (g)	carb (g)	fat (g)
Sanguinello					
TROPICANA	39		0.5	8.7	0
Summer Fruits Cordial					
diluted (100ml) BOTTLEGREEN		22	0	5.6	Tr
undiluted, organic ROCK'S	251		0.1	63	Tr
Summer Fruits Squash					
ROBINSONS	56		0.1	12.9	Tr
no added sugar ROBINSONS	9		0.1	1.1	Tr
Sunny Delight Drink					
apple & blackcurrant, each (200ml) PROCTER & GAMBLE		72	0.8	14.8	0.2
Caribbean, each (200ml) PROCTER & GAMBLE		69	0.8	14.8	0.2
Florida, each (200ml) PROCTER & GAMBLE		70	0.8	14.8	0.2
Tangerine Cordial					
undiluted, organic ROCK'S	257		0.2	64	Tr
Tomato Juice	14		0.8	3	Tr
BRITVIC	21		1	3.6	0.1
DEL MONTE	19		0.8	3.5	Tr
LIBBY	22		0.6	4.6	Tr
SCHWEPPES	30		0.8	7.2	0
Tropical Fruit Juice					
TROPICANA	45		0.5	10.6	0

Food Type	cal per 100g/ml	cal per portion	pro (g)	carb (g)	fat (g)
Tropical Squash					
undiluted, organic ROCK'S	221		0.1	55	Tr
V8					
pomegranate & cranberry					
juice CAMPBELL'S	38		0.3	9	0.1
tropical CAMPBELL'S	35		0.4	8.1	0.1
vegetable juice CAMPBELL'S	19		0.8	3.2	0.3
Water, flavoured					
all flavours	1		Tr	Tr	0
Smoothies					
Blackberries, Raspberries & Boysenberries Smoothie					
INNOCENT	44		0.6	13.1	Tr
Blackberry & Blueberry Smoothie					
TROPICANA	51		0.7	11.5	Tr
Carrots & Mangoes Smoothie					
INNOCENT	60		0.6	15.6	Tr
Cranberries & Raspberries Smoothie					
INNOCENT	46		0.6	12.8	Tr
Cranberry Smoothie					
OCEAN SPRAY	66		0.6	14.9	0

Food Type	cal per 100g/ml	cal per portion	pro (g)	carb (g)	fat (g)
Cranberry & Blackcurrant Smoothie					
OCEAN SPRAY	62		0.7	13.6	0.1
Cranberry & Raspberry Smoothie					
OCEAN SPRAY	58		0.7	12.7	0
ST CLEMENTS	55		0.6	12	0.2
Mango, Passionfruit & Pineapple Smoothie					
TROPICANA	52		0.7	11.6	Tr
Mango & Passionfruit Smoothie					
ST CLEMENTS	55		0.6	12.1	0.2
INNOCENT	56		0.5	14.8	0.3
Oranges, Mangoes & Pineapples Smoothie					
for kids, INNOCENT	55		0.6	13.7	0.1
Peaches & Passion Fruits Smoothie					
for kids, INNOCENT	58		0.6	15.2	Tr
Pineapples, Bananas & Coconuts Smoothie					
INNOCENT	69		0.8	14.9	1.3
Pomegranates, Blueberries & Blackcurrants Smoothie					
for kids, INNOCENT	53		0.3	13.8	Tr

Food Type	cal per 100g/ml	cal per portion	pro (g)	carb (g)	fat (g)
Strawberries & Bananas Smoothie					
INNOCENT	53		0.6	14.3	Tr
Strawberries, Blackberries & Raspberries Smoothie					
for kids, INNOCENT	46		0.5	12.4	Tr
Strawberry & Banana Smoothie					
ST CLEMENTS	61		0.8	13.4	0.2
Frijj Milkshakes					
banana, each (500ml) DAIRY CREST		305	17	50.5	4
chocolate, each (500ml)					
DAIRY CREST		385	19.5	63	7.5
strawberry, each (500ml)					
DAIRY CREST		325	18.5	52.5	4.5
Fizzy Drinks					
7 Up					
PEPSICO	41		0	10.7	0
cherry PEPSICO	39		0.1	10.2	0
free PEPSICO	1.9		0.1	0.1	0
Apple Juice Drink					
BRITVIC 55	46		0.1	11	0.1
Apple, Raspberry & Cranberry Juice Drink					
BRITVIC 55	40		0.1	9.4	0.1

Food Type	cal per 100g/ml	cal per portion	pro (g)	carb (g)	fat (g)
Bitter Lemon					
BRITVIC	45		0.5	9.8	0.1
SCHWEPPES	34		0	8.2	0
Slimline SCHWEPPES	2		Tr	0.1	0
Coca-Cola					
COCA-COLA	43		0	10.6	0
caffeine-free, diet COCA-COLA	0.4		0	0	0
cherry COCA-COLA	45		0	11.2	0
cherry, diet COCA-COLA	1		0	0	0
citrus zest, diet COCA-COLA	1		0	0	0
diet COCA-COLA	0.4		0	0	0
vanilla COCA-COLA	43		0	10.7	0
zero COCA-COLA	1		0	0	0
Cox's Apple Pressé					
BOTTLEGREEN	29		0	7.3	0
Cranberry & Orange Pressé					
BOTTLEGREEN	29		0	7.3	0
Cream Soda					
BARR	29		Tr	7.1	0
with twist of raspberry BARR	49		0	11.5	0
Dandelion & Burdock					
BARR	42		0	10.3	0
diet BARR	1		Tr	0.2	0

Food Type	cal per 100g/ml	cal per portion	pro (g)	carb (g)	fat (g)
Dr Pepper					
COCA-COLA	41.7		0	10.4	0
zero COCA-COLA	1		0	0	0
Elderflower Pressé					
BOTTLEGREEN	29		0	7.3	0
Fanta					
fruit twist COCA-COLA	53		Tr	13.6	0
lemon COCA-COLA	34		Tr	8.3	0
lemon, zero COCA-COLA	1.9		Tr	0.2	0
orange COCA-COLA	43		0	10.5	0
orange zero COCA-COLA	3.3		0	0.6	0
Ginger Ale, American	23		Tr	5.5	0
BRITVIC	38		0	9.2	0
Ginger Ale, Canada Dry					
SCHWEPPES	38		0	9	0
Ginger Beer					
IDRIS	35		Tr	8.5	0
Ginger & Elderflower Pressé					
BOTTLEGREEN	29		0	7.3	0
Irn Bru					
BARR	43		Tr	10.5	0
diet BARR	0.7		0	Tr	0
Lemonade					
bottled	22		Tr	5.8	0
SCHWEPPES	18		Tr	4.2	0

Food Type	cal per 100g/ml	cal per portion	pro (g)	carb (g)	fat (g)
Lemonade, Premium					
R WHITES	12		Tr	2.5	Tr
diet R WHITES	2		Tr	Tr	Tr
Lilt					
COCA-COLA	20		0	4.6	0
Lilt					
light COCA-COLA	4		0	0.6	0
Lucozade Glucose Drink					
GLAXO SMITHKLINE	70		Tr	17.9	0
apple GLAXO SMITHKLINE	70		Tr	17.2	0
lemon GLAXO SMITHKLINE	70		Tr	17	0
orange GLAXO SMITHKLINE	70		Tr	17.2	0
tropical GLAXO SMITHKLINE	70		Tr	17.3	0
wild berry GLAXO SMITHKLINE	70		Tr	17.1	0
Orange Juice Drink					
BRITVIC 55	49		0.3	11.3	0.1
Orange & Mango Pressé					
BOTTLEGREEN	29		0	7.3	0
Orangina					
BARR	42		0.1	10.2	0
light BARR	6		0.1	1.2	0
Pepsi					
PEPSICO	42		0	11	0
diet PEPSICO	0.4		0.1	0	0

Food Type	cal per 100g/ml	cal per portion	pro (g)	carb (g)	fat (g)
Pepsi Max					
PEPSICO	0.3		0.1	0	0
Pomegranate & Elderflower Pressé					
BOTTLEGREEN	29		0	7.3	0
Purdey's Multivitamin Fruit Drink					
BRITVIC	32		0.2	6.8	0.1
Red Bull					
energy RED BULL	45		0	11.3	0
sugar-free RED BULL	3		0	1	0
Schloer					
red grape SCHLOER	42		Tr	10.4	0
white grape SCHLOER	42		Tr	10.5	0
white grape & elderflower SCHLOER	37		Tr	9.2	0
white grape, mango & passionfruit SCHLOER	39		Tr	9.6	0
white grape, raspberry & cranberry SCHLOER	34		Tr	8.5	0
Sprite					
COCA-COLA	43		0	10.5	0
zero COCA-COLA	1.2		0	0	0
Tango					
apple BRITVIC	10		Tr	2.1	0

Food Type	cal per 100g/ml	cal per portion	pro (g)	carb (g)	fat (g)
cherry BRITVIC	11		0.1	2.4	0
citrus BRITVIC	10		0.1	2	Tr
orange BRITVIC	19		0.1	4.4	Tr
orange, low calorie BRITVIC	4		0.1	0.4	Tr
Tonic Water	33		0	8.8	0
SCHWEPPES	37		0	0	0
Slimline SCHWEPPES	2.5		0	0	0
Water, flavoured					
all flavours	1		Tr	Tr	0
Coffee & Tea					
Coffee					
infusion, 5 minutes, average		2	0.2	0.3	Tr
instant, powdered	75		14.6	4.5	Tr
Alta Rica					
NESCAFÉ	98		13.8	10	0.3
decaffeinated NESCAFÉ	98		13.8	10	0.3
Blend 37					
NESCAFÉ	97		14	10	0.1
Cappio					
caffé latte KENCO	415		12.5	63.5	12
original cappuccino KENCO	395		10.5	66.5	9.9
unsweetened cappuccino KENCO	405		9.5	67	10.5
Cappuccino					
NESCAFÉ	443		11.7	60.3	17.4
café caramel NESCAFÉ	421		9.2	64.6	14.1

Food Type	cal per 100g/ml	cal per portion	pro (g)	carb (g)	fat (g)
café vanilla NESCAFÉ	430		9.3	64.6	14.9
decaffeinated NESCAFÉ	427		11.6	62.6	14.6
decaffeinated, unsweetened NESCAFÉ	475		10.4	52.9	24.6
double choca mocha NESCAFÉ	408		9.2	68	11
mocha NESCAFÉ	417		8.5	66.6	13.1
skinny NESCAFÉ	318		23.6	43.9	4.4
unsweetened NESCAFÉ	462		15	47.3	23.8
Chamomile Herbal Tea					
caffeine-free CELESTIAL SEASONINGS	0		0	0	0
Coffeemate					
per 6.5g tsp NESCAFÉ		36	0.2	3.7	2.2
virtually fat-free, per 6.5g tsp NESCAFÉ		26	0.2	5.5	0.4
Echinacea & Rasperry Tea					
TWININGS	2		Tr	Tr	Tr
Espresso					
instant NESCAFÉ	104		15.2	10	0.4
Gold Blend					
all varieties NESCAFÉ	63		7	36	0.2
Green Tea					
TWININGS	1		Tr	0.2	0.3
Ice Tea					
lemon LIPTON'S	28		0	6.7	0
peach LIPTON'S	29		0	6.9	0

Drinks (Non-alcoholic)

Food Type	cal per 100g/ml	cal per portion	pro (g)	carb (g)	fat (g)
Latte					
NESCAFÉ	494		14.5	45.7	28.5
Irish Cream NESCAFÉ	424		8.2	65.2	14.1
Nescafé					
all varieties NESCAFÉ	63		7	9	0.2
Nestea Lemon					
COCA-COLA	32		0	7.7	0
Redbush Tea					
TWININGS	3		Tr	Tr	0.3
Tea					
infusion, black	Tr		0.1	Tr	Tr
PG TIPS	Tr		0.1	Tr	0
extra strong TETLEY	1		0	0.3	0
White Tea, China Pearl					
decaffeinated CELESTIAL					
SEASONINGS	0		0	0	0
Hot/Milk Drinks					
Aero Hot Chocolate					
as sold NESTLÉ	414		8.7	69.2	11.2
mint, as sold NESTLÉ	414		8.3	70.8	10.8
Banana Nesquik					
as sold NESTLÉ	394		0	24.3	0
fresh, each (250ml) NESTLÉ		175	8.1	26.7	3.9
Beef Concentrate Drink					
as prepared (12g) BOVRIL		22	4.7	0.6	0.1

Food Type	cal per 100g/ml	cal per portion	pro (g)	carb (g)	fat (g)
Chicken Concentrate Drink					
as prepared (12g) BOVRIL		16	1.2	2.3	0.2
Chocolate Nesquik					
as sold NESTLÉ	367		4.2	21.6	3.2
fresh, each (250ml) NESTLÉ		190	8.6	28.6	4.3
Cocoa Powder	312		18.5	11.5	21.7
fairtrade	330		23.1	10.5	21.7
Bournville CADBURY	330		23.1	10.5	21.7
organic GREEN & BLACK	350		23.6	13.6	22.3
Drinking Chocolate					
powder	373		5.4	79.7	5.8
made with 200ml					
semi-skimmed milk		73	3.6	10.9	2
made with 200ml whole milk		90	3.5	10.7	4
CADBURY	370		6.3	73.3	5.9
CAFÉDIRECT	372		8.9	65.1	8.4
Galaxy Instant Hot Chocolate Drink					
as sold MARS	412		7	68.7	12.1
4 heaped tsps with water MARS		115	2	19.2	3.4
Highlights					
CADBURY	360		17.5	43.3	13.2
fudge CADBURY	355		16.8	50.7	9.6
mint CADBURY	365		17.4	44.3	13.1
orange CADBURY	360		18.5	41	13.5

Food Type	cal per 100g/ml	cal per portion	pro (g)	carb (g)	fat (g)
Horlicks					
with 200ml semi-skimmed milk GLAXO SMITHKLINE		181	9.5	27.2	4.2
Horlicks Extra Light Chocolate					
per sachet (11g), made with water GLAXO SMITHKLINE		33	n/a	n/a	0.7
Horlicks Extra Light Malt					
per sachet (11g), made with water GLAXO SMITHKLINE		35	n/a	n/a	0.7
dreamy vanilla, per sachet (11g), made with water GLAXO SMITHKLINE		35	n/a	n/a	0.7
heavenly amaretto, per sachet (11g), made with water GLAXO SMITHKLINE		35	n/a	n/a	0.7
Horlicks Light Malt					
made with 32g powder & water GLAXO SMITHKLINE		115	4.8	22	0.8
Horlicks Light Malt Chocolate					
made with 32g powder & water GLAXO SMITHKLINE		121	2.9	23	1.9
Hot Chocolate					
instant, as sold CADBURY	425		10.9	64.2	14
instant, as sold GALAXY	411		7	68.7	12.1
instant, as sold SKINNY COW	370		19.7	39.3	14.6

Food Type	cal per 100g/ml	cal per portion	pro (g)	carb (g)	fat (g)
mint, instant, as sold					
SKINNY COW	370		19.5	39.9	14.4
organic, as sold GREEN & BLACK	374		9.1	63.5	9.3
Hot Chocolate, Maltesers					
instant, as sold AIMIA FOODS	374		9.1	63.5	9.3
Options					
Belgian chocolate, as prepared					
with 11g powder		37	1.2	5.3	1.1
cracking hazelnut, as prepared					
with 11g powder		40	1	6.3	1.2
mint madness, as prepared					
with 11g powder		41	1.3	6.2	1.1
outrageous orange, as					
prepared with 11g powder		41	1.3	6.1	1.1
wickedly white, as prepared					
with 11g powder		45	1.2	7	1.4
Ovaltine					
powder OVALTINE	370		7.3	80	1.9
made up with 200ml					
semi-skimmed milk		191	8.6	30.1	3.8
light	396		16.8	62.7	8.5
light, made with 25g					
powder & water		99	4.2	15.7	2.1
Ovaltine Chocolate					
OVALTINE	362		8	75.7	3

Food Type	cal per 100g/ml	cal per portion	pro (g)	carb (g)	fat (g)
made with 200ml					
semi-skimmed milk		190	8.8	29.1	4.1
light	358		9	67.1	5.6
light, made with 25g powder					
& water		72	1.8	13.4	1.2
Ovaltine White					
made with 200ml					
semi-skimmed milk		195	8	31.3	4.2
Strawberry Nesquik					
as sold NESTLÉ	393		0	25	0
fresh, each (250ml) NESTLÉ		170	8.2	26	4

Food Type	cal per 100g	cal per portion	pro (g)	carb (g)	fat (g)
Eggs					
Eggs, chicken					
raw, whole	151		12.5	Tr	11.2
raw, white only	36		9	Tr	Tr
raw, yolk only	339		16.1	Tr	30.5
boiled	147		12.5	Tr	10.8
fried, in vegetable oil	179		13.6	Tr	13.9
poached	147		12.5	Tr	10.8
Eggs, duck					
raw, whole	163		14.3	Tr	11.8

Food Type

Food Type	cal per 100g	cal per portion	pro (g)	carb (g)	fat (g)
Fast Food					
McDonald's					
Apple Pie					
each		240	2	29	13
Bacon, Egg & Cheese Bagel					
each		480	22	49	21
Bacon & Egg McMuffin					
each		340	20	26	17
double, each		395	25	26	21
Belgian Bliss Brownie					
each		390	5	43	22
Big Mac					
each		490	28	41	24
Cheeseburger					
each		295	16	31	12
double		440	28	32	23
Deli Chicken & Bacon					
brown roll, each		485	21	58	19
Deli Chicken & Bacon					
brown roll, with cheese, each		555	26	60	23
Dips					
BBQ, per portion		50	0	11	0
smokey BBQ, per portion		85	0	19	1
sour cream & chive, per portion		160	0	2	17
sweet chilli, per portion		125	0	29	1

Food Type	cal per 100g	cal per portion	pro (g)	carb (g)	fat (g)
sweet curry, per portion		50	0	11	1
sweet & sour, per portion		50	0	11	0
Chicken Legend with Cool Mayo					
per portion		550	30	61	21
Chicken Legend with Spicy					
Tomato Salsa					
per portion		515	30	67	14
Chicken McNuggets					
6 nuggets		250	14	20	14
Chicken Selects					
5 pieces		610	35	43	33
Crispy Chicken Salad					
per portion		270	23	18	12
with bacon, per portion		325	28	19	15
Filet-O-Fish					
each		350	15	36	16
Fish Finger					
portion		195	13	16	9
French Fries					
large, per portion		460	5	60	23
medium, per portion		330	3	42	16
small, per portion		230	2	30	11
Fruit Bag					
per portion		40	0	10	0

Food Type	cal per 100g	cal per portion	pro (g)	carb (g)	fat (g)
Garden Salad					
per portion		10	1	2	0
Grilled Chicken Salad					
per portion		115	18	6	2
with bacon, per portion		165	23	6	5
Hamburger					
each		250	14	30	8
Hash Browns					
per portion		130	1	14	7
Little Italian					
each		290	16	30	12
M					
each		545	34	43	26
McChicken Sandwich					
each		385	16	44	16
Mayo Chicken					
each		315	13	37	12
Milkshake					
banana, medium, each		425	9	72	11
chocolate, medium, each		415	9	67	12
strawberry, medium, each		420	9	70	11
vanilla, medium, each		420	9	70	11
Mozzarella Dippers					
per portion		265	11	23	14

Food Type	cal per 100g	cal per portion	pro (g)	carb (g)	fat (g)
Muffin, Blueberry					
low-fat, each		300	6	63	3
Muffin, Double Chocolate					
each		425	7	56	19
Quarter Pounder with Cheese					
each		490	31	37	25
Salsa Snack Wrap					
each		345	13	32	18
Sausage, Egg & Cheese Bagel					
each		560	28	50	28
Sausage & Egg McMuffin					
each		420	25	27	23
double, each		560	36	27	34
Sundae, Strawberry					
each		360	4	70	7
Sundae, Toffee					
each		350	5	62	9
Toasted Deli Chicken Salad					
brown roll, each		365	21	57	6
brown roll, with cheese, each		430	26	59	10
Toasted Deli Spicy Veggie					
brown roll, each		540	13	92	13
brown roll, with cheese, each		605	19	93	17

Food Type	cal per 100g	cal per portion	pro (g)	carb (g)	fat (g)
Toasted Deli Sweet Chilli Chicken					
brown roll, each		605	30	85	16
brown roll, with cheese, each		670	35	86	21
Wimpy					
Bacon in a bun					
each		212	13.1	30.5	3.5
Bacon & Egg in a Bun					
each		301	19.9	30.5	10.5
BBQ Burger					
each		647	33.8	61.7	30.2
Bender in a Bun					
each		383	14.7	37	19.9
with cheese, each		424	17.2	37.7	23.1
BLT in a Bun					
each		216	13.4	31.4	3.6
Cheeseburger					
each		312	16.6	55	20
Chicken Chunks with Chips					
each		740	24.2	69	41.9
Chicken in a Bun					
each		408	15.4	41.4	20.8
Chicken Salad					
gourmet, each		254	42.4	10.4	4.3
hot 'n spicy, each		267	15.1	22.5	13.2

Food Type	cal per 100g	cal per portion	pro (g)	carb (g)	fat (g)
Classic					
each		337	19.7	31.6	15.1
with cheese, each		379	22.2	32.2	31
Classic Bacon Cheeseburger					
each		406	26.4	32.4	18.9
Classic Bacon Grill					
each		722	36.8	44.8	45.3
Classic Kingsize					
each		552	36.9	32.2	31
Fish Salad					
each		389	16.5	35.3	21.3
Great Wimpy Breakfast					
each		779	42.8	59.7	41.2
Haddock, Chips & Peas					
portion		676	20.6	66.8	38.1
Halfpounder					
each		842	54.8	36.7	53.7
Hamburger					
each		270	14.2	30.7	10.5
Hash Browns					
portion	93		1.2	10.8	7.8
Jacket Potato with Grated Cheese					
each		973	43.1	90.7	51.3
Paninis					
ham & cheese, each		596	34.3	64.7	22.2

Food Type	cal per 100g	cal per portion	pro (g)	carb (g)	fat (g)
Pork Rib					
portion		455	24.3	39.9	22
Quarterpounder					
each		538	30	36	31.3
with cheese		579	32.4	36.7	34.4
Sausage, Egg & Chips					
each		597	22	42.4	38.8
Spicy Beanburger					
each		594	12.8	72	29
Toasted Tea Cake & Butter					
each		237	5	34.9	9
Wimpy Classic Grill					
each		755	35	44.3	51
Wimpy Club					
each		640	42.3	60.3	26.1
Burger King					
Angus					
each		550	28	41	29
double, each		791	50	41	46
Apple Pie					
portion		330	3	49	14
Big Breakfast Butty					
with ketchup, each		845	42	50	51
BK Bacon Butty					
with ketchup, each		386	18	39	17

Food Type	cal per 100g	cal per portion	pro (g)	carb (g)	fat (g)
Cheeseburger					
each		311	16	28	14
Chicken Bites					
14 bites		282	21	13	16
Chicken Royale					
each		569	24	47	31
with cheese, each		661	29	49	38
Egg & Cheese Butty					
with ketchup, each		449	17	39	24
Flame-grilled Chicken Salad					
each		99	14	6	1
with French dressing, each		106	14	7	1
French Fries					
large, per portion		388	4	53	18
regular, per portion		305	3	42	14
small, per portion		204	2	28	9
Garden Salad					
per portion		35	2	6	Tr
Hamburger					
each		266	14	28	10
Hash Browns					
regular, per portion		333	3	31	22
Ocean Catch					
each		486	17	40	28

Food Type	cal per 100g	cal per portion	pro (g)	carb (g)	fat (g)
Onion Rings					
regular, per portion		325	6	43	14
Strawberry Cheesecake					
portion		346	6	27	24
Veggie Bean Burger					
each		547	19	74	22
Whopper					
each		631	29	48	35
with cheese, each		718	34	49	42
Pizza Hut					
BBQ Delux					
medium pan, per slice		276	12.6	30.9	11.3
Breaded Chicken Sticks					
portion		368	34	22	16
Caesar Salad					
chicken, portion		296	20	20.4	14.8
classic, portion		366	14	25.2	23.1
Cheesy Bites					
per slice, chicken supreme		309	16.7	41.8	9.6
per slice, hot n spicy		331	16	42.7	12.5
per slice, meat feast		387	19.8	43.1	16.2
per slice, vegetable supreme		312	14.5	44.6	10
Chicken Supreme					
medium pan, per slice		251	11.2	30.5	9.9

Food Type	cal per 100g	cal per portion	pro (g)	carb (g)	fat (g)
Dips					
BBQ, portion		34	0.4	8.2	0
Sour Cream & Chive, portion		82	0.3	1.1	1.1
Sweet Chilli, portion		48	0.1	9.2	0.1
Farmhouse Medium Pan					
per slice		242	11.3	28.6	10.4
Garlic Bread with Cheese					
portion		568	29.8	35.6	34
Garlic Ciabatta					
portion		820	23	109.8	32.1
Goats' Cheese Melt Medium Pan					
per slice		273	10.2	30.6	13.6
Hawaiian Medium Pan					
per slice		245	11.1	31.2	9.8
Hot 'n' Spicy Medium Pan					
per slice		237	10.7	27.2	10.6
Lasagne					
portion		589	27.1	59.8	26.7
Margherita Medium Pan					
per slice		256	11.2	29.5	11.4
Meat Feast Medium Pan					
per slice		294	13.7	31.5	13.9
Mediterranean Meat Deluxe Medium Pan					
per slice		245	11.5	27.6	11.2

Food Type	cal per 100g	cal per portion	pro (g)	carb (g)	fat (g)
Nachos					
portion		669	17.1	67.1	40.2
Pepperoni Feast					
medium pan, per slice		297	13.4	27.9	15.9
Potato Wedges					
portion		382	5.5	54.1	16.1
Seafood Lovers					
medium pan, per slice		233	9.6	27.9	10.4
Spinach & Ricotta Cannelloni					
portion		568	25.1	53.1	27.5
Stuffed Crust					
per slice, margherita		318	18	40.6	11.3
per slice, meat feast		376	20.5	42.6	15.8
per slice, vegetable supreme		308	16.9	14.5	43.5
Supreme					
medium pan, per slice		310	12.6	32.3	15.7
Supreme, Super					
medium pan, per slice		323	14.4	28.9	18.5
Tagliatelle alla Carbonara					
portion		548	22.4	41.6	32.4
Texas BBQ Chicken Wings					
portion		355	34.1	5.7	21.8
The Italian					
per slice, margherita		204	8.7	28.4	7
per slice, meat feast		257	12.9	29.8	10.9

Food Type	cal per 100g	cal per portion	pro (g)	carb (g)	fat (g)
per slice, vegetable supreme		196	8.2	30.5	6.1
Vegetable Supreme					
medium pan, per slice		263	10.8	32.7	11.2
Vegetarian Hot One					
medium pan, per slice		234	9.7	30.6	9.9
Domino's Pizza					
American Hot					
medium, per slice		194	10.5	22.1	7
Cheese & Tomato					
medium, per slice		162	8.5	21.2	4.8
Chicken Kickers					
per portion		182	16.4	14	6.7
Chicken Strippers					
per portion		224	16.2	12.9	11.8
Coleslaw					
per portion		160	1.2	6.4	14.4
Dips					
BBQ, per portion		23	0	5.5	0.1
Sweet Chilli, per portion		30	0.1	7.1	0.1
Full House					
medium, per slice		250	14.1	24.3	10.7
Garlic Mushrooms					
per portion		133	4.5	18.5	4.5
Garlic Pizza Bread					
per slice		274	16.6	30.6	9.5

Food Type	cal per 100g	cal per portion	pro (g)	carb (g)	fat (g)
Hawaiian					
medium, per slice		192	11.9	22	6.3
Hot & Spicy					
medium, per slice		179	9.5	22.1	5.9
Meatball Mayhem					
medium, per slice		262	10.9	32.8	9.7
Meateor					
medium, per slice		257	11.1	30.9	9.8
Mighty Meaty					
medium, per slice		218	12.8	21.8	9
Pepperoni Passion					
medium, per slice		244	14.7	21.6	10.7
Potato Wedges					
per portion		149	2.4	20.8	6.2
Sizzler					
medium, per slice		248	12.8	27.4	9.7
Tandoori Hot					
medium, per slice		176	10.5	22	5
Texas BBQ					
medium, per slice		223	11.1	30.3	6.3
Vegetarian Supreme					
medium, per slice		170	8.8	22.6	4.9
Fish & Chips					
Chips					
fried in oil	239		3.2	30.5	12.4

Food Type	cal per 100g	cal per portion	pro (g)	carb (g)	fat (g)
Cod					
in batter, fried	247		16.1	11.7	15.4
Plaice					
in batter, fried	257		15.2	12	16.8
Rock Salmon/Dogfish					
in batter, fried	295		14.7	10.3	21.9
Skate					
in batter, fried	168		14.7	4.9	10.1
Boots Shapers					
Apple, Strawberry & Kiwi in Greek Yogurt					
per pack		83	1.8	13	n/a
Blackcurrant Yogurt Granola					
each		188	6.7	28	5.5
Blueberry Yoghurt					
each		104	5.6	17	1.5
Blueberry & Yoghurt Nougat Bar					
each		89	0.4	13	3.6
Carrot & Sugar Snap Pea Snack					
per pack		32	1.4	6.2	0.2
Chargrilled Mediterranean Vegetable Ciabatta					
each		267	11	49	3.3

Food Type	cal per 100g	cal per portion	pro (g)	carb (g)	fat (g)
Cheese & Celery Sandwich					
per pack		324	n/a	45	7.3
Cheese & Onion Crispy Discs					
per pack		93	1.3	13	3.9
Chicken Arrabiata Pasta					
per pack		264	10	44	4.9
Chicken Caesar Salad					
per pack		191	19	16	5.6
Chicken Fajita Wrap					
per pack		284	22	39	4.5
Chicken Tikka Sandwich					
per pack		282	23	41	2.9
Chicken & Basil Pesto Ciabatta					
each		339	25	44	7.1
Chicken & Pesto Sandwich					
per pack		329	23	40	8.8
Chocolate Mint Nougat Bar					
each		83	0.6	16	3.2
Cloudy Apple Drink					
sparkling, per pack		27	n/a	5.5	0
Cool Mint Nougat & Chocolate Bar					
per portion		83	n/a	16	3.2
Cranberry Juice Drink					
per pack		40	0	9.6	0

Food Type	cal per 100g	cal per portion	pro (g)	carb (g)	fat (g)
Crayfish & Rocket Salad					
per pack		74	10	1.8	2.9
Crispy Bacon Bites					
per pack		93	1.8	13	3.8
Crispy Chocolate & Orange Bar					
each		93	0.8	17	2.6
Crunchy Apple & Juicy Grape Fruit Bag					
per pack		46	0.1	0.1	0.3
Crunchy Carrot Snack					
per pack		28	n/a	6	0.2
Crunchy Onion Rings					
per pack		61	0.3	7.4	3.3
Egg Mayonnaise & Cress Sandwich					
per pack		291	16	39	7.6
Egg, Tomato & Spinach Baguette					
each		250	n/a	37	6.4
Flatbreads, Chicken Tikka					
each		263	18	37	4.9
Flatbreads, Greek Salad					
each		225	11	34	4.9
Flatbreads, Tex Mex Chicken & Salsa					
each		263	19	38	3.6

Food Type	cal per 100g	cal per portion	pro (g)	carb (g)	fat (g)
Fruit Smoothies, 100%					
strawberry & raspberry, each		121	n/a	11	0.9
Ham, Soft Cheese & Sunblush					
Tomato Sandwich					
per pack		265	17	37	5.2
Honey Mustard Chicken					
Pasta Salad					
per pack		350	21	54	5.4
Houmous & Carrot Sandwich					
per pack		323	15	42	10
Houmous & Chargrilled					
Vegetable Wrap					
per pack		250	15	3.8	4.6
Lemon & Lime Drink					
sparkling, per pack		9	0	0.3	0
Lemon & Yoghurt Nougat Bar					
each		91	n/a	17	2.5
Lemonade, Cloudy					
sparkling, per pack		7	0	0.5	0
Lemonade, Still					
per pack		15	0.1	1.8	0
Melon, Kiwi, Blueberry &					
Pomegranate					
per portion		60	1.6	13	0.2

Food Type	cal per 100g	cal per portion	pro (g)	carb (g)	fat (g)
Melon & Grape					
per portion		75	1.2	17	0.2
Morrocan Chicken Couscous					
per pack		310	13	48	7.7
Orange Drink					
vitamin enriched, per pack		31	0.3	5.3	Tr
Orange & Raspberry Fruit Crush					
each		122	1.3	28	0.6
Pineapple, Melon & Probiotic Yogurt Snack					
per pack		58	3.8	10	0.3
Pineapple Wedges with Mango & Coconut Dip					
per pack		89	1.4	18	1.4
Potato Tubes					
per pack		65	0.9	8.9	2.9
Prawn Mayonnaise Sandwich					
per pack		297	18	42	6.7
Prawn Spirals					
per pack		70	0.5	9.6	3.3
Raspberry Granola Yoghurt					
each		188	6.7	28	5.5
Raspberry Yoghurt					
each		95	5.4	15	1.5

Food Type	cal per 100g	cal per portion	pro (g)	carb (g)	fat (g)
Raspberry & Mango Drink					
sparkling, per pack		5	n/a	0	0
Raspberry & White Chocolate Cookies					
Mini, per pack		136	n/a	22	4.3
Ready Salted Crispy Discs					
per pack		93	1.1	13	3.9
Red Thai Chicken Wrap					
per pack		255	19	34	4.8
Rhubarb Yoghurt					
each		94	5.6	14	1.6
Salmon & Cucumber Sandwich					
per pack		287	n/a	43	3.8
Salt & Vinegar Chipsticks					
per pack		99	1.3	14	4.5
Salt & Vinegar Crispy Discs					
per pack		92	1	13	3.9
Salt & Vinegar Spirals					
per pack		70	0.5	9	3.5
Salted Pretzels					
mini, per pack		95	2.5	20	0.5
Salted Tubes					
per pack		65	0.9	8.9	2.9

Food Type	cal per 100g	cal per portion	pro (g)	carb (g)	fat (g)
Sliced Melon Snack Pack					
per pack		25	0.6	5.4	0.1
Sliced Pineapple Snack Pack					
per pack		35	0	0	0.2
Sour Cream & Chives Crispy Discs					
per pack		97	n/a	13	4
Sour Cream & Chives Mini Pretzels					
per pack		93	2.8	18	0.7
Strawberry Cereal Bar, Prebiotic					
each		85	0.9	15	2.2
Strawberry Nougat Bar					
each		84	n/a	17	3
Strawberry Yoghurt					
each		100	n/a	16	1.5
Strawberry & Kiwi Drink					
still, per bottle		5	0.1	0	Tr
Summer Fruits Drink					
sparkling, per carton		6	Tr	Tr	Tr
Sunblush Tomato, Soft Cheese & Roasted Vegetable Sandwich					
per pack		270	18	39	4.6
Superfood Salad					
per pack		41	0.8	6.3	1.3

Food Type	cal per 100g	cal per portion	pro (g)	carb (g)	fat (g)
Sushi Rolls					
per portion		234	8.9	43	3
Sushi Rolls, Deluxe					
per portion		354	12	68	3.5
Sweet Chilli Chicken Wrap		279	19	43	3.5
Thai Chilli Crunchies					
per pack		96	1.4	13	4.2
Tomato & Basil Chicken Pasta					
per pack		425	24	49	15
Tuna Crunch					
each		221	12	23	3.4
Tuna Sandwich					
per pack		285	n/a	40	4.7
Tuna & Cucumber Sandwich					
per pack		285	n/a	40	4.7
Tuna & Sweetcorn Pasta Salad					
per pack		306	n/a	0.5	2.9
Turkey, Stuffing & Cranberry Sandwich					
per pack		328	24	54	2.2
Tzatziki Chicken Sandwich					
per pack		286	n/a	39	4.4
Vegetable Pakora Sandwich					
per pack		301	12	47	7.2

Food Type	cal per 100g	cal per portion	pro (g)	carb (g)	fat (g)
Vegetarian Sushi					
per pack		206	4.6	43	1.5
Watermelon Wedges with Strawberry & Raspberry Dip					
per pack		86	0.1	21	0.1
Yogurt & Mint Multigrain Snack					
per pack		80	1.3	10	3.8
Pret A Manger					
All Day Breakfast Sandwich					
each		560	29.4	48.9	27.5
Avocado & Herb Salad Wrap					
each		461	12.1	35.5	30.2
Avocado & Pesto Sandwich					
each		457	11.5	40.6	26.4
Beech-smoked BLT Sandwich					
each		493	21.1	38.2	28.8
Brie, Tomato & Whole-leaf Basil Baguette					
each		432	17.9	49	18.3
Carrot Card Box Cake					
per pack		402	4.5	45.9	22.3
Cheddar, Roast Tomatoes & Pickle Bloomer					
each		648	27.1	60.3	24.1

Food Type	cal per 100g	cal per portion	pro (g)	carb (g)	fat (g)
Chef's Italian Chicken Salad					
each		322	21.3	9.9	24.1
Chicken Avocado Sandwich					
each		456	21.8	39.7	23.7
Chicken Caesar Baguette					
each		517	25.3	49.5	23.9
Chicken Valentino Sandwich					
each		516	26.6	40.2	25.2
Chicken & Fresh Pesto Salad					
each		328	25	3.1	22.8
Chocolate Brownie					
each		267	2.8	28.6	15.7
Classic Super Club Sandwich					
each		548	29.1	38	31.5
Croissant					
each		324	6.6	31.6	18.9
Croissant, Almond					
each		365	8.8	34.9	21.1
Croissant, Chocolate					
each		406	7.5	42.9	24.3
Deluxe Sushi					
each		311	13.8	54.6	3.1
Double Berry Muffin					
each		470	6.3	57.9	23.8

Food Type	cal per 100g	cal per portion	pro (g)	carb (g)	fat (g)
Drinks					
cappuccino, each (12oz)		106	5.9	7.6	5.8
hot chocolate, each (12oz)		309	10.2	39.4	12.4
latte, each (12oz)		194	10.5	13.2	11.2
mocha, with chocolate, each (12oz)		243	9.5	25.8	11.4
Free-range Egg & Bacon Sandwich					
each		511	25.2	36.9	29.3
Hoisin Duck Wrap					
each		433	20.1	43.7	20.1
Italian Prosciutto Artisan Baguette					
each		636	26.8	67.7	28.5
Jalapeno Chicken Hot Wrap					
each		433	33.2	42.8	14.6
Mature Cheddar & Pret Pickle Sandwich					
each		588	25.7	45.6	33.9
Pain au Raisin					
each		306	5.2	42.3	12.7
Roasted Red Peppers & Swiss Sandwich					
each		473	17.1	40.5	26.9

Food Type	cal per 100g	cal per portion	pro (g)	carb (g)	fat (g)
Simply Ham & Mustard Mayo Sandwich					
each		467	27	37.8	23.1
Skipjack Tuna Baguette					
each		484	21.1	47.9	22.9
Skipjack Tuna Sandwich					
each		442	20	38.1	22.7
Slim Pret					
all day breakfast, each		306	12.8	23.4	17.9
beech-smoked BLT, each		248	10.5	19.1	14.4
chicken avocado, each		228	10.8	19.9	11.9
chicken valentino, each		258	13.3	20.1	12.6
classic super club, each		274	14.5	19	15.8
Italian prosciutto artisan baguette, each		318	13.4	33.8	14.2
mature cheddar & pret pickle, each		294	12.9	22.8	17
Skipjack tuna baguette, each		242	10.6	24	11.5
Skipjack tuna sandwich, each		234	11.2	18.8	12.7
wild crayfish & rocket, each		185	8.1	18.9	8.6
Spicy Falafel Melt					
each		460	20.2	51.4	19.3
Vegetarian Sushi					
each		277	6.5	49.9	5.4

Food Type	cal per 100g	cal per portion	pro (g)	carb (g)	fat (g)
Wild Crayfish & Rocket Sandwich					
each		370	16.2	37.8	17.2
Wild Poached Salmon & Horseradish Sandwich					
each		379	21.4	40.2	14.3
Yoghurt & Pecan Muffin					
each		521	10.4	49.3	31.6
Starbucks					
Apple & Cinnamon Muffin					
each		413	6.2	58.1	18.9
Belgian Chocolate Brownie					
each		317	3.7	40	16
BLT Sandwich					
each		527	17.4	40.9	32.6
Blueberry Muffin					
each		449	7.2	58.2	23
Blueberry Muffin, Skinny					
each		361	6	72.4	6
British Chicken & Green Pesto Panini					
each		352	25	43	8.9
British Chicken & Red Pesto Pasta Salad					
each		390	21.5	45.9	13.3

Food Type	cal per 100g	cal per portion	pro (g)	carb (g)	fat (g)
Cheese & Marmite Panini					
each		297	16.5	34.9	10.1
Chocolate Cake, Fairtrade					
each		330	7.6	28.5	19.8
Chocolate Caramel Shortbread					
each		320	2.3	36.6	18.2
Cinnamon Swirl					
each		432	9.8	81	7.7
Croissant, Almond					
each		465	8.5	53	24.4
Croissant, Butter					
each		279	4.8	27.7	16.5
Drinks					
brewed coffee, tall, black, each	4		0.5	0	0.1
brewed tea, tall, black, each	0		0	0	0
caffe Americano, tall, black, each	11		0.7	2	0
caffe misto, tall, whole milk, each	97		5.3	7	5.2
cappuccino, tall, whole milk, each	108		5.9	9	5.6
frappuccino blended coffee, light, tall, each	91		4.4	18	0.7
frappuccino blended coffee, tall, each	184		3.9	37	2.4

Food Type	cal per 100g	cal per portion	pro (g)	carb (g)	fat (g)
hot chocolate, tall, whole milk					
and whipped cream, each		433	11.6	45	26.1
latte, tall, whole milk, each		176	9.5	14	5.3
mocha, tall, whole milk and					
whipped cream, each		290	10.2	33	15.5
Tazo chai tea latte, whole					
milk, each		194	5.5	33	5
Egg & Bacon Panini					
each		305	16.3	36	10.4
Fruit Salad					
each		67	1	16.1	0.3
Houmous with Foccacia Sticks					
dip pot, each		258	8.1	26.2	13.7
Houmous & Roasted					
Vegetable Wrap					
each		415	12.7	59.8	13.7
Mature Cheddar & Pickle					
Sandwich					
each		491	17.9	43.4	27.3
Mini Ham & Cheese Toastie					
each		345	19	40.2	11.8
Mozzarella & Slow Roast					
Tomato Panini					
each		461	20	48.7	20.7

Food Type	cal per 100g	cal per portion	pro (g)	carb (g)	fat (g)
Oak Smoked Salmon & Rocket Sandwich					
each		360	20.7	34.1	15.6
Sicilian Lemon Cupcake					
each		350	2.6	44.2	18
Tuna & Three Bean Salad					
each		335	25.2	32.2	12
Tuna Mayonnaise Sandwich					
each		333	16.8	40.7	11.4
Tzatziki with Vegetable Sticks					
dip pot, each		73	2.8	6.8	3.9

Food Type	cal per 100g	cal per portion	pro (g)	carb (g)	fat (g)
Fish & Seafood					
Fish & Seafood					
Anchovies					
canned in oil, drained	191		25.2	0	10
Basa					
skinless fillets YOUNG'S	77		16.4	0	1.3
Cockles					
boiled	53		12	Tr	0.6
pickled PARSONS	82		13.8	4.1	1.1
Cod					
baked fillets	96		21.4	Tr	1.2
dried, salted, boiled	138		32.5	0	0.9
poached fillets	94		20.9	Tr	1.1
steaks, grilled	95		20.8	Tr	1.3
Cod Roe					
hard, fried	202		20.9	3	11.9
pressed JOHN WEST	110		14	5	4
see also: ROE					
Coley Fillets					
steamed	105		23.3	0	1.3
Crab					
boiled	128		19.5	Tr	5.5
canned in brine, drained	77		18.1	Tr	0.5
canned in brine, drained PRINCES	76		16.7	2	0.1

Food Type	cal per 100g	cal per portion	pro (g)	carb (g)	fat (g)
Crayfish Medley					
LYONS SEAFOODS	81		14.3	3.1	1.3
Crayfish Tails					
cooked, peeled BIG PRAWN CO.	51		10.1	1	0.7
cooked, peeled LYONS SEAFOODS	61		13.1	1	0.5
Eels					
jellied	98		8.4	Tr	7.1
Haddock					
in crumbs, frozen, fried	196		14.7	12.6	10
smoked, steamed	101		23.3	0	0.9
steamed	89		20.9	0	0.6
skinless and boneless, frozen					
YOUNG'S	81		18	Tr	6
Halibut					
grilled	121		25.3	0	2.2
Herring					
raw	190		17.8	0	13.2
fried, flesh only	234		23.1	1.5	15.1
grilled	181		20.1	0	11.2
grilled, flesh only	199		20.4	0	13
Kippers					
raw	229		17.5	0	17.7
grilled	255		20.1	0	19.4
fillets, smoked YOUNG'S	198		15.5	0.4	15

Food Type	cal per 100g	cal per portion	pro (g)	carb (g)	fat (g)
Lemon Sole					
goujons, baked	187		16	14.7	14.6
goujons, fried	374		15.5	14.3	28.7
steamed	91		20.6	0	0.9
Lobster					
boiled	119		22.1	0	3.4
dressed JOHN WEST	105		13	2	5
Mackerel					
grilled	239		20.8	0	17.3
raw	220		18.7	0	16.1
smoked	354		18.9	0	30.9
in olive oil, canned JOHN WEST	329		17.9	Tr	28.6
Mussels					
boiled	87		17.2	Tr	2
in white wine sauce	86		8.5	5	3.6
pickled PARSONS	97		16.7	1.3	2.8
smoked, canned in sunflower oil JOHN WEST	230		16	10	14
Octopus					
chunks, canned in olive oil PALACIO DE ORIENTE	148		24	5	4
smoked, canned in sunflower oil JOHN WEST	230		16	10	14
Pilchards					
canned in tomato sauce	126		18.8	0.7	5.4

Food Type	cal per 100g	cal per portion	pro (g)	carb (g)	fat (g)
fillets, canned in sunflower oil					
PRINCES	233		26.3	Tr	14.2
fillets, canned in tomato sauce					
PRINCES	136		20	1.5	5.6
Plaice					
in batter, fried	257		15.2	12	16.8
in crumbs, fried	228		18	8.6	13.7
goujons, baked	304		8.8	27.7	18.3
goujons, fried	426		8.5	27	32.3
steamed	93		18.9	0	1.9
Prawns					
boiled	99		22.6	0	0.9
boiled, weighed in shells	41		8.6	0	0.7
boiled, in shell LYONS SEAFOODS	64		14.7	0.1	0.6
Greenland YOUNG'S	69		15.4	0.1	0.8
in shell, whole, cooked,					
Atlantic LYONS SEAFOODS	64		14.7	0.1	0.6
king, cooked & peeled	76		14.9	1.4	1.2
king, raw & peeled	74		16.3	0.5	0.8
king, warm water, cooked &					
peeled BIRDS EYE	65		14.7	0.1	0.6
tiger, whole, raw	65		14	0	1
Roe					
cod, hard, fried	202		20.9	3	11.9
cod, soft JOHN WEST	84		12	Tr	4

Food Type	cal per 100g	cal per portion	pro (g)	carb (g)	fat (g)
herring, soft, fried	244		21.1	4.7	15.8
Salmon					
fillet, grilled	169		25.7	Tr	7.3
fillet, chilled YOUNG'S	213		24	0	13
fillet, frozen YOUNG'S	177		20.6	0.6	10.3
pink, canned, in brine, drained	153		23.5	0	6.6
pink, wild, canned JOHN WEST	155		23	Tr	7
red, wild, canned JOHN WEST	168		24	Tr	8
red, wild, canned PRINCES	166		18.9	0	10
smoked	142		25.4	0	4.5
smoked JOHN WEST	185		22.2	0.5	10.5
smoked YOUNG'S	156		23.5	0	6.9
steamed	194		21.8	0	11.9
Sardines					
canned in oil, drained	220		23.3	0	14.1
canned in sunflower oil JOHN WEST	255		21.7	Tr	15.4
canned in tomato sauce	162		17	1.4	9.9
canned in tomato sauce JOHN WEST	164		17	1.5	10
Scallops					
frozen without shells YOUNG'S	91		18.3	3.5	0.5
Seafood Selection					
chilled YOUNG'S	88		17.1	2.8	0.9

Food Type	cal per 100g	cal per portion	pro (g)	carb (g)	fat (g)
Shrimps					
canned, drained	94		20.8	Tr	1.2
frozen, without shells	73		16.5	Tr	0.8
Skate					
battered, fried	168		14.7	4.9	10.1
fried in butter	199		17.9	4.9	12.1
skinned skate wings	81		19	0	0.5
Squid					
chunks, in ink sauce PALACIO DE ORIENTE	228		13	3.6	18
Swordfish					
grilled	139		22.9	0	5.2
Trout					
brown, steamed, flesh only	135		23.5	0	4.5
rainbow, grilled	135		21.5	0	5.4
Tuna					
smoked fillet, canned in olive oil JOHN WEST	191		26.7	Tr	9.3
steak, fresh	136		23.7	0	4.6
Tuna, chunks/steaks, drained					
canned in brine	99		23.5	0	0.6
canned in brine JOHN WEST	108		26.2	Tr	0.3
canned in brine PRINCES	105		25	0	0.5
canned in oil	189		27.1	0	9
canned in sunflower oil JOHN WEST	161		28.2	Tr	5.4

Food Type	cal per 100g	cal per portion	pro (g)	carb (g)	fat (g)
canned in sunflower oil					
PRINCES	167		25	0	7.4
in spring water PRINCES	105		25	0	0.5
Whelks					
boiled	89		19.5	Tr	1.2
Whitebait					
in flour, fried	525		19.5	5.3	47.5
Whiting					
in crumbs, fried	191		18.1	7	10.3
steamed, flesh only	92		20.9	0	0.9
Winkles					
boiled	72		15.4	Tr	1.2

For Fish Pâté and Spreads see:

SAVOURY SPREADS AND PASTES

Breaded, Battered or in Sauces

Food Type	cal per 100g	cal per portion	pro (g)	carb (g)	fat (g)
Cod Fillets					
in batter, fried	247		16.1	11.7	15.4
in crumbs, frozen, fried	235		12.4	15.2	14.3
in natural crumb	180		11.1	17.9	7.4
in parsley sauce, frozen,					
boiled	84		12	2.8	2.8
Chip Shop YOUNG'S	224		10.4	12.7	14.6
Chip Shop, chunky breaded					
YOUNG'S	187		12.7	13.6	9.1

Food Type	cal per 100g	cal per portion	pro (g)	carb (g)	fat (g)
in crunch crumb BIRDS EYE	181		12.9	14.1	8.1
Cod Steak					
in batter, fried in oil	247		16.1	11.7	15.4
in crumbs, fried in oil	235		12.4	15.2	14.3
in butter sauce YOUNG'S	77		11.3	2.1	2.6
in parsley sauce YOUNG'S	70		10.1	2.5	2.2
Fish Bakes					
Broccoli & Cheese BIRDS EYE	132		12.2	3.6	7.6
Mixed Vegetable BIRDS EYE	102		12	4.8	3.9
Fish Cakes					
fried	218		8.6	16.8	13.4
Chip Shop YOUNG'S	200		7.8	21.1	9.4
Fish Cakes, Cod					
in crunch crumb BIRDS EYE	187		11.8	15.7	8.5
Fish Cakes, Haddock					
chilled YOUNG'S	227		9	15	14.6
Fish Fillets					
Chip Shop, in salt & vinegar					
batter YOUNG'S	216		10.5	13	13.5
Fish Fingers					
fried in oil	233		13.5	17.2	12.7
grilled	214		15.1	19.3	9
in crispy batter BIRDS EYE	240		10.9	16.6	14.4
Megas BIRDS EYE	202		13.4	20.5	7.4
Omega 3 BIRDS EYE	183		12.8	15.1	7.9

Food Type	cal per 100g	cal per portion	pro (g)	carb (g)	fat (g)
value BIRDS EYE	176		12.5	15.5	7.1
Fish Fingers, Cod Fillet					
fried in oil	238		13.2	15.5	14.1
grilled	200		14.3	16.6	8.9
BIRDS EYE	182		12.8	15.1	7.8
Fish Fingers, Haddock Fillet					
BIRDS EYE	188		14.3	15.1	7.8
Fish Fingers, Salmon Fillet					
BIRDS EYE	225		13.2	21.7	9.5
Fish Steaks					
in butter sauce YOUNG'S	77		10.2	2.8	2.8
in parsley sauce YOUNG'S	70		10.1	2.5	2.2
Haddock					
in crumbs, fried in oil	196		14.7	12.6	10
Haddock Fillets					
Chip Shop YOUNG'S	234		11	14.9	14.6
Chip Shop, chunky breaded					
YOUNG'S	185		12.5	14.5	8.5
in beer batter BIRDS EYE	211		14.6	13.7	10.9
with a cheese & chive sauce					
YOUNG'S	102		13	1.7	4.8
Haddock Mornay					
chilled YOUNG'S	123		11.6	2.2	7.5
Hake in a Cheese & Chive Sauce					
chilled YOUNG'S	126		11.8	1.3	8.6

Food Type	cal per 100g	cal per portion	pro (g)	carb (g)	fat (g)
Plaice					
in batter, fried in oil	257		15.2	12	16.8
in crumbs, fried, fillets	228		18	8.6	13.7
Pollock Fillets					
in crispy batter BIRDS EYE	239		11.4	23.5	11
in crunchy breadcrumbs					
BIRDS EYE	209		11.8	23	7.7
Prawn Cocktail	245		7	7	21
YOUNG'S	115		7.8	7.4	6.4
Salmon Fillets					
Alaskan, with a watercress					
sauce YOUNG'S	98		14.1	1.8	3.8
Atlantic, in a white wine sauce					
YOUNG'S	180		10.5	1.1	14.8
lemon & pepper YOUNG'S	242		16.7	0.9	19.1
wild, in garlic & herb crumb					
top BIRDS EYE	133		16.8	6.6	4.4
Scampi in Breadcrumbs					
frozen, fried	237		9.4	20.5	13.6
wholetail BIRDS EYE	207		8.6	20.9	9.9
wholetail YOUNG'S	202		9.6	22.4	9.1
Scampi Kievs					
YOUNG'S	241		10.7	19.4	13.4
Seafood Sticks					
YOUNG'S BLUECREST	112		7.8	18.3	0.8

Food Type	cal per 100g	cal per portion	pro (g)	carb (g)	fat (g)
Tuna with a Twist					
with a lime & black pepper dressing JOHN WEST	156		15.6	2.8	9.2
Whiting					
in crumbs, fried	191		18.1	7	10.3
Meals					
Admiral's Pie					
YOUNG'S	95		4.1	10.9	3.9
Chargrilled Tuna Steak in Soy & Ginger Dressing					
PRINCES	118		26.1	2.3	0.5
Chargrilled Tuna Steak in Tomato & Basil Dressing					
PRINCES	118		26.1	2.3	0.5
Fish Fillet Dinner					
YOUNG'S	94		6.2	8.2	4.1
Fish Pastry Pie					
YOUNG'S	262		7.4	16.9	18.3
Fish Pie					
WEIGHTWATCHERS	72		4.4	9.6	1.8
Healthy Options BIRDS EYE	75		3.9	11.8	1.4
in butter sauce ROSS		90	4.7	9.8	3.6
in parsley sauce ROSS		94	5	11.2	3.2
Fish & Vegetable Pie					
YOUNG'S	131		6.4	9.6	7.4

Food Type	cal per 100g	cal per portion	pro (g)	carb (g)	fat (g)
Fisherman's Crumble					
YOUNG'S	109		4	12	5
Fisherman's Pie					
YOUNG'S	95		4.1	10.9	3.9
King Prawn Makhani with Basmati Rice					
chilled YOUNG'S	92		4.7	12.2	2.8
Mariner's Pie					
YOUNG'S	105		5	12	4.1
Mediterranean Fish Bake with Mozzarella Crumb					
YOUNG'S	116		9.4	5.7	6.2
Mediterranean Fish Gratin					
chilled YOUNG'S	114		10.1	4.7	6.1
Ocean Crumble					
low fat YOUNG'S	81		5.1	10.6	2
Ocean Pie					
WEIGHTWATCHERS	70		4.5	9.6	1.5
YOUNG'S	103		5.8	9.6	4.6
Salmon Crumble					
YOUNG'S	102		5.4	11.1	4
Salmon en Croute, Atlantic					
chilled YOUNG'S	264		10.3	15.3	17.9
Salmon Fillet Dinner					
YOUNG'S	84		6.7	7.9	2.8

Food Type	cal per 100g	cal per portion	pro (g)	carb (g)	fat (g)
Salmon Pie					
YOUNG'S	117		6.4	11.9	4.9
Salmon & Broccoli Pie					
YOUNG'S	109		6.3	9.6	5.1
Salmon & Broccoli Wedge Melt					
WEIGHTWATCHERS	93		5.1	10.6	3.3
Salmon & Penne Pasta					
chilled YOUNG'S	146		10.5	10.5	6.9
Tuna Light Lunches					
French style, each JOHN WEST	221		18.9	22.6	6.2
tomato salsa, each JOHN WEST	180		20	18.7	2.8
Vintage Cheddar Fish Bake					
YOUNG'S	105		9.5	6.8	4.5

Food Type	cal per 100g	cal per portion	pro (g)	carb (g)	fat (g)
Flour & Baking					
Flour					
Barleycorn Bread Flour					
organic DOVES FARM	334		8.2	71.1	1.9
Buckwheat Flour					
organic DOVES FARM	335		11.9	65.4	2.9
Cornflour	354		0.6	92	0.7
BROWN & POLSON	343		0.6	83.6	0.7
organic DOVES FARM	351		0.3	86.3	0.6
Chapati Flour					
medium NATCO	327		10.7	68.8	2
Gram Flour					
organic DOVES FARM	336		12.8	60	5
Ground Rice					
WHITWORTHS	349		7.7	77.7	0.8
Kamut Bread Flour					
organic DOVES FARM	325		15	60.9	2.3
Malthouse Bread Flour					
organic DOVES FARM	325		12.3	64.5	2
Rice Flour					
organic DOVES FARM	357		8.4	75.9	2.2
Rye Flour, whole	335		8.2	75.9	2
organic DOVES FARM	304		7.6	64.1	1.9

Food Type	cal per 100g	cal per portion	pro (g)	carb (g)	fat (g)
Sauce Flour					
per 15g CARR'S		50.9	1.5	11	0.2
Soya Flour					
full fat	447		36.8	23.5	23.5
low fat	352		45.3	28.2	7.2
Spelt Flour					
white, organic DOVES FARM	342		13.8	67.2	2
wholegrain, organic					
DOVES FARM	330		13.3	63.6	2.5
Wheat Flour					
brown	324		12.6	68.5	2
white, breadmaking	337		11	70	1.4
white, plain	336		10	71	1.3
white, self-raising	343		11	72	1.2
wholemeal, plain	308		14	58	2.2
00 premium grade MCDOUGALL'S	332		11	69.3	1.4
self-raising sponge flour					
MCDOUGALL'S	351		8	76.7	1.4
Pastry					
Filo	311		9	62	3
uncooked JUS-ROL	234		8.1	52.1	2.7
Flaky					
cooked	564		5.6	46	41

Food Type	cal per 100g	cal per portion	pro (g)	carb (g)	fat (g)
Pastry Mix					
gluten-free MRS CRIMBLE'S	574		6	66.3	31.6
Puff					
uncooked	419		5	30	31
Puff, Block					
uncooked JUS-ROL	401		5.6	31.2	28.6
Puff, Ready Rolled					
uncooked JUS-ROL	401		5.6	30.2	28.6
Shortcrust					
cooked	524		6.6	54.3	32.6
Shortcrust, All Butter					
uncooked JUS-ROL	431		6.3	40.1	27.3
Shortcrust, Block					
uncooked JUS-ROL	462		7	38.7	31
Shortcrust, Flan Case					
uncooked JUS-ROL	468		6.1	38.5	34.4
Shortcrust, Mix					
MCDOUGALLS	478		8	53	26
Shortcrust, Ready Rolled					
uncooked JUS-ROL	460		7.1	39.1	30.6
Vol-au-Vent Cases					
uncooked, frozen JUS-ROL	401		5.6	30.2	28.6
Wholemeal					
cooked	501		8.9	44.6	33.2

Food Type	cal per 100g	cal per portion	pro (g)	carb (g)	fat (g)
Baking Agents					
Baking Powder	163		5.2	37.8	0
Yeast, Baker's					
compressed	53		11.4	1.1	0.4
Yeast, Baker's					
dried	169		35.6	3.5	1.5
Bread Mixes					
Cheese & Onion Bread Mix					
WRIGHT'S BAKING	233		9.3	45.3	2.2
Ciabatta Bread Mix					
WRIGHT'S BAKING	343		14.2	71	3
Garlic & Rosemary Focaccia Bread Mix					
WRIGHT'S BAKING	329		9.4	43.7	13
Granary Bread Mix					
HOVIS	231		9	38.6	4.5
Malty Bread Mix					
WRIGHT'S BAKING	234		9.2	44.3	2.3
Mixed Grain Bread Mix					
WRIGHT'S BAKING	322		13.1	66	4
Mrs Crimble's Bread Mix					
gluten free MRS CRIMBLE'S	217		2.5	44.4	3.3
Naan Bread Mix					
SHARWOOD'S	370		11.8	66.8	6.2

Food Type	cal per 100g	cal per portion	pro (g)	carb (g)	fat (g)
Parmesan & Sun-Dried Tomato Bread Mix					
WRIGHT'S BAKING	229		9	44.4	1.7
Scofa Bread Mix					
WRIGHT'S BAKING	214		7.5	44	1.1
White Bread Mix					
CARR'S	334		13.1	67.6	1.2
HOVIS	228		10.8	33.6	5.7
WRIGHT'S BAKING	240		9.3	46.8	1.8
Wholemeal Bread Mix					
CARR'S	313		14.6	59	2.1
HOVIS	220		9.4	36.1	4.2
organic DOVES FARM	221		9.1	35.6	4.7
Sweet Mixes					
Batter Mix					
MCDOUGALL'S	316		9.5	37.7	14.1
Butterfly Tops Mix					
GREEN'S	407		4.2	62.8	15.4
Carmelle Mix					
GREEN'S	89		3.3	15.1	1.7
Carrot Cake Mix					
WRIGHT'S BAKING	341		6.7	47.3	14.1
Cheesecake Mix					
GREEN'S	320		4.5	39.5	16

Food Type	cal per 100g	cal per portion	pro (g)	carb (g)	fat (g)
Choc Orange Muffin Mix					
GREEN'S	322		4.5	49.6	11.7
Chocolate Chip Cake Mix					
organic DOVES FARM	392		6.6	41.8	22.1
Chocolate Fudge Cake Mix					
JANE ASHER	363		3.3	50.2	18
WRIGHT'S BAKING	362		6.6	45.3	17.7
Chocolate Mousse Torte Dessert Mix					
DR OETKER	304		4.8	23.6	21.2
Coconut Cake Mix					
JANE ASHER	377		3.7	48.6	18.6
Crumble Topping Mix					
MCDOUGALL'S	462		6.5	67.9	18.3
Egg Custard Mix					
no bake GREEN'S	88		3.9	13.7	1.9
Ginger Cake Mix					
WRIGHT'S BAKING	321		5.8	49	11.4
Lemon Drizzle Cake Mix					
JANE ASHER	338		3.2	50	15.3
Lemon Drizzle Muffin Mix					
WEIGHTWATCHERS	235		7.1	51.5	3.6
Lemon Meringue Crunch Mix					
GREEN'S	274		1.8	43.7	10.2

Food Type	cal per 100g	cal per portion	pro (g)	carb (g)	fat (g)
Lemon Pie Filling Mix					
GREEN'S	88		0.4	19.1	1.1
Lively Lemon Muffin Mix					
GREEN'S	337		4	52.5	12.4
Madeira Cake Mix					
WRIGHT'S BAKING	349		5.9	48.2	14.4
New York Style Baked Cheesecake Dessert Mix					
DR OETKER	342		5.7	29.4	22
Oat & Raisin Cookies Mix					
GREEN'S	443		6.1	65.7	32.4
Pancake Mix					
GREEN'S	202		5.1	31.1	6.3
Toffee Cake Mix					
WRIGHT'S BAKING	305		5.8	41.2	13
Victoria Sandwich Mix					
GREEN'S	390		3.2	57.4	16.4
Sundries					
Cherries					
glacé BILLINGTON'S	313		0.3	79.6	0.1
Chocolate, 72% Cook's					
organic, GREEN & BLACK	566		9.6	31.2	44.7
Chocolate Chips, Milk					
fairtrade, organic SUPERCOOK	512		5.8	65.5	26.2

Food Type	cal per 100g	cal per portion	pro (g)	carb (g)	fat (g)
Chocolate Drops, Plain					
organic DOVES FARM	505		5.7	58.9	27.4
Chocolate Flakes, Milk					
organic DOVES FARM	507		7.8	56.7	27.7
Ginger, Crystallised					
HOLLAND & BARRETT	330		0.3	82	0.1
Lemon Juice					
fresh	7		0.3	1.6	Tr
bottled JIF	24		0.5	2	Tr
Lime Juice					
bottled JIF	27		n/a	0.7	Tr
Marzipan					
golden or white	426		6	69	14
natural DR OETKER	428		6.6	67.5	14.6
ready rolled SUPERCOOK	434		6.5	67.7	15.2
select DR OETKER	443		9.2	56.2	20.2
Mincemeat	274		0.6	62.1	4.3
with madeira wine & almonds	291		1.6	59.4	5.2
ROBERTSON'S	275		0.7	61.5	2.9
Mixed Peel	231		0.3	59.1	0.9
Pie Filling					
fruit	77		0.4	20.1	Tr
apple & blackberry HARTLEY'S	86		0.2	22.2	0.1
black cherry HARTLEY'S	99		0.4	24.3	0.1
bramley apple HARTLEY'S	85		0.2	21.1	0.1

Food Type	cal per 100g	cal per portion	pro (g)	carb (g)	fat (g)
Regal Icing					
white, ready rolled SUPERCOOK	398		0	87.5	5.6
Royal Icing					
SILVER SPOON	396		0.7	98.2	Tr
Fairtrade TATE & LYLE	395		1.4	97.5	0
Vanilla Pod					
whole SCHWARTZ	235		n/a	25	15

Food Type	cal per 100g	cal per portion	pro (g)	carb (g)	fat (g)

Fruit

Fresh & Canned Fruit

Apples, Cooking

Food Type	cal per 100g	cal per portion	pro (g)	carb (g)	fat (g)
flesh only	35		0.3	8.9	0.1
stewed with sugar	74		0.3	19.1	0.1
stewed without sugar	33		0.3	8.1	0.1
Apples, Eating					
flesh only	45		0.4	11.2	0.1
flesh & skin, raw	47		0.4	11.8	0.1
Apricots					
flesh & skin, raw	31		0.9	7.2	0.1
canned in juice	34		0.5	8.4	0.1
canned in syrup	63		0.4	16.1	0.1
canned in syrup DEL MONTE	68		0.4	15.5	0.2
Bananas					
peeled	95		1.2	23.2	0.3
Blackberries	25		0.9	5.1	0.2
canned in fruit juice	32		0.6	7	0.2
stewed with sugar	56		0.7	13.8	0.2
stewed without sugar	21		0.8	4.4	0.2
Blackcurrants	28		0.9	6.6	Tr
canned in juice	34		0.6	8	Tr
canned in syrup	72		0.7	18.4	Tr
stewed with sugar	58		0.7	15	Tr

Food Type	cal per 100g	cal per portion	pro (g)	carb (g)	fat (g)
Breadfruit					
canned, drained	66	0.6	16.4	0.2	
Cherries					
flesh & skin	48	0.9	11.5	0.1	
canned in syrup	71	0.5	18.5	Tr	
Cherries, black					
canned in heavy syrup	86	0.8	20.3	0.2	
Clementines					
flesh only	37	0.9	8.7	0.1	
Coconut					
creamed	669	6	7	68.8	
desiccated	604	5.6	6.4	62	
creamed BLUE DRAGON	182	1.9	2.3	18.3	
creamed block BLUE DRAGON	667	10	1	67	
creamed block PATAK	600	5.6	6.4	62	
desiccated WHITWORTHS	606	5.6	6.4	62	
milk BLUE DRAGON	194	2.1	4.2	18.7	
milk, reduced fat AMOY	21	1.2	3.8	0.1	
Cranberries					
raw OCEAN SPRAY	55	0	13	0	
Damsons					
flesh & skin	38	0.5	9.6	Tr	
stewed with sugar	74	0.4	19.3	Tr	
Dates					
flesh & skin	124	1.5	31.3	0.1	

Food Type	cal per 100g	cal per portion	pro (g)	carb (g)	fat (g)
block WHITWORTHS	288		3.3	68	0.2
chopped HUMDINGER	303		2.2	72.2	0.5
stoned CRAZY JACK'S	297		2.1	71	0.5
Figs	122		0.4	7.2	Tr
Fruitini Mixed Fruit Pieces					
in juice DEL MONTE	59		0.4	14	0.1
Fruit cocktail					
canned in juice	29		0.4	7.2	Tr
canned in juice DEL MONTE	55		0.4	12.6	0.1
canned in juice JOHN WEST	50		0.3	12	0.1
canned in syrup	57		0.4	14.8	Tr
canned in syrup DEL MONTE	63		0.4	15	0.1
Fruit Compote					
apple and berry, organic					
YEO VALLEY	75		0.4	18.2	0.1
orchard fruits, organic YEO VALLEY	67		0.4	16.3	0.1
summer fruits, organic YEO VALLEY	62		0.6	14.6	0.1
Fruit Express					
peach pieces in juice DEL MONTE	59		0.5	13.8	0.1
peach & pear in juice DEL MONTE	59		0.4	13.8	0.1
pineapple chunks in juice					
DEL MONTE	56		0.4	13	0.1
tropical fruit pieces in juice DEL MONTE					

Fruit

Food Type	cal per 100g	cal per portion	pro (g)	carb (g)	fat (g)
Fruit Salad	44		0.7	10.2	0.1
tropical NATURE'S FINEST	60		2.5	11.9	Tr
Gooseberries					
canned in syrup HARTLEY'S	73		0.6	17	0.2
Grapefruit					
flesh only	30		0.8	6.8	0.1
canned segments in juice					
DEL MONTE	48		0.6	10.5	Tr
Grapes					
black/white, seedless	60		0.4	15.4	0.1
Greengages					
flesh & skin	34		0.5	8.6	Tr
stewed with sugar	107		1.3	26.9	0.1
Guavas	26		0.8	5	0.5
canned in syrup	60		0.4	15.7	Tr
Jackfruit	88		1.3	21.4	0.3
canned, drained	104		0.5	26.3	0.3
Kiwi fruit					
peeled	49		1.1	10.6	0.5
Lemons					
whole	19		1	3.2	0.3
Lychees	58		0.9	14.3	0.1
canned in syrup	68		0.4	17.7	Tr
canned in syrup BLUE DRAGON	59		0.5	14	0

Food Type	cal per 100g	cal per portion	pro (g)	carb (g)	fat (g)
canned in syrup JOHN WEST	72		0.4	17.7	Tr
canned in syrup PREMIER GOLD	68		0.4	17.7	Tr
Mandarin oranges					
canned in juice	32		0.7	7.7	Tr
canned in juice DEL MONTE	45		0.6	10	0.1
canned in juice NATURE'S FINEST	36		0.6	12.4	0.3
canned in syrup	52		0.5	13.4	Tr
canned in syrup LA DORIA	54		0.5	13	Tr
Mangos					
flesh only	57		0.7	14.1	0.2
canned in syrup	57		0.7	14.1	0.2
slices, canned in syrup					
BLUE DRAGON	93		0.3	22.6	0.1
slices, canned in syrup JOHN WEST	65		0.3	16	Tr
Melon					
flesh only, cantaloupe-type	19		0.6	4.2	0.1
flesh only, galia	24		0.5	5.6	0.1
flesh only, honeydew	28		0.6	6.6	0.1
flesh only, watermelon	31		0.5	7.1	0.3
Nectarines					
flesh & skin	40		1.4	9	0.1
Oranges					
flesh only	37		1.1	8.5	0.1
Papaya, Red					
spears, in juice NATURE'S FINEST	45		0.3	10.4	Tr

Fruit

Food Type	cal per 100g	cal per portion	pro (g)	carb (g)	fat (g)
Passionfruit					
flesh & pips only	36		2.6	5.8	0.4
Paw-Paw					
flesh only	36		0.5	8.8	0.1
canned in juice	65		0.2	17	Tr
Peaches	33		1	7.6	0.1
canned in natural juice	39		0.6	9.7	Tr
canned in natural juice DEL MONTE	49		0.5	11.2	0.1
canned in syrup	55		0.5	14	Tr
canned in syrup DEL MONTE	65		0.4	15.5	0.1
Pears	40		0.3	10	Tr
canned in natural juice	33		0.3	8.5	Tr
canned in natural juice DEL MONTE	45		0.3	10.5	0.1
canned in syrup	50		0.2	13.2	Tr
canned in syrup DEL MONTE	58		0.2	14	0.1
Pineapple					
flesh only	41		0.4	10.1	0.2
canned in natural juice	47		0.3	12.2	Tr
canned in natural juice DEL MONTE	69		0.4	15.5	0.1
canned in syrup	64		0.5	16.5	Tr
Plums	36		0.6	8.8	0.1
canned in syrup	59		0.3	15.5	Tr
red, canned in syrup JOHN WEST	73		0.3	18	Tr
Prunes					
canned in juice	79		0.7	19.7	0.2

Food Type	cal per 100g	cal per portion	pro (g)	carb (g)	fat (g)
canned in juice DEL MONTE	91		0.6	21.7	0.1
canned in syrup	90		0.6	23	0.2
Raspberries	25		1.4	4.6	0.3
stewed with sugar	48		0.9	11.5	0.1
canned in juice JOHN WEST	32		0.9	6.7	0.2
canned in syrup	88		0.6	22.5	0.1
canned in syrup HARTLEY'S	75		0.8	17.5	0.2
frozen	27		1.2	4.9	0.3
Rhubarb	7		0.9	0.8	0.1
canned in syrup	31		0.5	7.6	Tr
canned in syrup HARTLEY'S	31		0.5	7.3	Tr
stewed with sugar	48		0.9	11.5	0.1
stewed without sugar	7		0.9	0.7	0.1
frozen	8		0.9	0.8	0.2
Satsumas					
flesh only	36		0.9	8.5	0.1
Strawberries	27		0.8	6	0.1
canned in syrup	65		0.5	16.9	Tr
Summer Fruits					
canned in syrup HARTLEY'S	71		0.5	17.2	0.1
Tangerines					
flesh only	35		0.9	8	0.1
Tropical Fruits					
in juice DEL MONTE	53		0.3	12.6	Tr

Food Type	cal per 100g	cal per portion	pro (g)	carb (g)	fat (g)
Watermelon					
flesh only	31		0.5	7.1	0.3
Dried Fruit					
Apple Crisps, FruitaBu					
KELLOGG'S	356		2	86	0.5
with natural blackcurrant					
KELLOGG'S	356		2	86	0.5
with natural strawberry					
KELLOGG'S	356		2	86	0.5
Apple Rings					
dried JULIAN GRAVES	270		0.9	65.9	0.3
Apricots					
ready to eat	158		4	36.5	0.6
dried, whole JULIAN GRAVES	296		3.7	68.9	0.6
Banana Chips					
dried JULIAN GRAVES	540		1.5	66.0	30.0
Craisins					
dried cranberries OCEAN SPRAY	319		0.1	76.6	1.4
with mixed berries OCEAN SPRAY	321		1.5	76.5	1
with mixed nuts & seeds OCEAN SPRAY	445		7.9	55.4	21.3
Cranberries					
HOLLAND & BARRETT	343		0.4	85	0.2
sweetened JULIAN GRAVES	343		0.4	84.9	0.4

Food Type	cal per 100g	cal per portion	pro (g)	carb (g)	fat (g)
Currants	267		2.3	67.8	0.4
dried JULIAN GRAVES	284		2.3	67.8	0.4
Dates					
dried, flesh & skin	270		3.3	68.0	0.2
dried, stoneless JULIAN GRAVES	287		3.3	68.0	0.2
dried, stoneless WHITWORTHS	287		3.3	68.0	0.2
Exotic Fruit Mix					
WHITWORTHS	271		2.4	64.1	0.6
Figs					
dried	227		3.6	52.9	1.6
dried, JULIAN GRAVES	267		3.3	63.9	0.9
Goji Berries					
HOLLAND & BARRETT	292		2.7	67.7	0.4
WHITWORTH	283		12.3	57.7	0.3
Mixed Fruit					
dried	268		2.3	68.1	0.4
Pineapple					
chunky pieces HOLLAND & BARRETT	347		0.1	84.1	Tr
diced & crystallised					
JULIAN GRAVES	358		0.6	87.6	0.6
Prunes					
canned in juice	79		0.7	19.7	0.2
canned in syrup	90		0.6	23.0	0.2
ready to eat	141		2.5	34	0.4
ready to eat, pitted JULIAN GRAVES	268		2.2	63.9	0.4

Food Type	cal per 100g	cal per portion	pro (g)	carb (g)	fat (g)
whole, pitted HOLLAND & BARRETT	160		2.8	38.4	0.5
Raisins					
seedless	272		2.1	69.3	0.4
chilean flame, JULIAN GRAVES	333		3.1	79.2	0.5
seedless JULIAN GRAVES	333		3.1	79.2	0.5
seedless SUN MAID	304		3	71.4	Tr
Snack Fruit Surprise					
HOLLAND & BARRETT	314		2.1	64.5	5
Strawberry Fruit Winders					
KELLOGG'S	389		0.2	79	8
Strawberry & Apple Fruit Winders					
KELLOGG'S	389		0.2	79	8
Strawberry & Blackcurrant Fruit Winders					
KELLOGG'S	389		0.2	79	8
Sultanas	275		2.7	69.4	0.4
JULIAN GRAVES	292		2.7	69.4	0.04

Food Type	cal per 100g	cal per portion	pro (g)	carb (g)	fat (g)
Jams, Marmalades & Sweet Spreads					
Jams, Marmalades & Honey					
Apricot Fruit Spread					
organic MERIDIAN FOODS	145		0.5	35.8	Tr
Apricot Jam					
Best HARTLEY'S	244		0.4	60.6	0
no-bits HARTLEY'S	256		0.3	63.7	0
Tiptree WILKIN & SONS	268		Tr	67	Tr
reduced sugar STREAMLINE	193		0.3	48	Tr
Black Cherry Jam					
Best HARTLEY'S	244		0.4	60.6	0
reduced sugar STREAMLINE	198		0.7	48	0.2
Blackberry Jam					
Best HARTLEY'S	244		0.4	60.5	0.1
Blackberry Jelly					
Tiptree WILKIN & SONS	268		Tr	67	Tr
Blackcurrant Conserve					
Tiptree WILKIN & SONS	268		Tr	67	Tr
Blackcurrant Fruit Spread					
organic MERIDIAN FOODS	133		0.6	32.6	Tr
Blackcurrant Jam					
Best HARTLEY'S	244		0.4	60.6	0
no-bits HARTLEY'S	256		0.2	63.8	0

Food Type	cal per 100g	cal per portion	pro (g)	carb (g)	fat (g)
reduced sugar STREAMLINE	198		0.6	48	0.4
Blackcurrant & Apple Jam					
smooth HARTLEY'S	196		0.3	48.7	0
Blueberry Fruit Spread, Wild					
no added sugar ST DALFOUR	228		0.5	56	0.2
organic MERIDIAN FOODS	150		0.7	36.8	Tr
Blueberry Jam					
Best HARTLEY'S	244		0.3	60.6	1
Bramble Preserve, Seedless					
MACKAYS	266		0.3	66	0
Cherry & Berry Fruit Spread					
organic MERIDIAN FOODS	138		0.7	33.7	Tr
Country Berry Conserve					
BAXTERS	243		0.5	60	0.1
Cranberry & Orange Fruit Spread					
organic MERIDIAN FOODS	134		0.5	32.9	Tr
Damson Jam					
Best HARTLEY'S	244		0.2	60.8	0
Fig Royale Fruit Spread					
no added sugar ST DALFOUR	231		0.8	56	0.4
Gooseberry Jam					
Tiptree WILKIN & SONS	268		Tr	67	Tr
Grapefruit Fruit Spread					
MERIDIAN FOODS	148		0.3	36.0	Tr

Food Type	cal per 100g	cal per portion	pro (g)	carb (g)	fat (g)
Honey					
clear, Hungarian acacia	305		0.4	76.4	0
clear CHIVERS	307		0.4	76.4	Tr
clear GALES	307		0.4	76.4	Tr
comb	281		0.6	74.4	4.6
organic, fine blossom WHOLE EARTH	302		0.3	75.1	0
organic, Maya wildflower					
WHOLE EARTH	302		0.4	75.1	0
set	306		0.4	76	0
set, New Zealand clover	305		0.4	76.4	0
Lemon Curd	282		0.6	62.7	4.9
GALES	293		0.7	61.4	4.9
MACKAYS	293		1.2	60.8	5
Tiptree WILKIN & SONS	334		2.1	49.9	14.3
Marmalade	261		0.1	69.5	0
Golden Shred ROBERTSON'S	253		0.2	62.3	Tr
Golden Shredless ROBERTSON'S	254		0.2	62.5	Tr
lemon BAXTERS	260		0.1	65	Tr
lemon ROSE'S	252		0.2	62.7	0.1
lemon, Silver Shred ROBERTSON'S	253		0.2	61.6	Tr
lemon & lime ROSE'S	260		0.2	64.8	0
lime, fine cut ROSE'S	264		0.1	65.9	0
orange, Dundee MACKAYS	255		0.2	63.6	0
orange, English Traditional					
DUERR'S	261		0.2	65	0

Food Type	cal per 100g	cal per portion	pro (g)	carb (g)	fat (g)
orange, fine cut DUERR'S	261		0.2	65	Tr
orange, fine cut ROSE'S	252		0.2	62.8	0
orange, lemon & grapefruit					
BAXTERS	261		0.3	65	Tr
orange, Olde English HARTLEY'S	276		0.3	68.7	0
orange, Oxford FRANK COOPER'S	272		0.4	67.6	0
orange, thick, reduced sugar					
STREAMLINE	191		0.3	47.1	0.2
orange, thin, Seville BAXTERS	261		0.3	65	Tr
orange & lemon MACKAYS	254		0.2	63.4	0
orange & lemon with ginger					
MACKAYS	254		0.2	63.4	0
Spanish grapefruit DUERR'S	261		0.2	65	Tr
three fruit MACKAYS	254		0.2	63.2	0
Morello Cherry Fruit Spread					
organic MERIDIAN FOODS	122		0.7	29.1	Tr
Orange & Ginger Fruit Spread					
no added sugar ST DALFOUR	254		0.2	63	0.1
Peach Jam					
reduced sugar, STREAMLINE	191		0.2	47.5	Tr
Pineapple Jam					
Best HARTLEY'S	244		0.2	60.7	0.1
Pineapple & Ginger Fruit Spread					
MERIDIAN FOODS	148		0.3	36	Tr

Food Type	cal per 100g	cal per portion	pro (g)	carb (g)	fat (g)
Raspberry Conserve					
BAXTERS	245		0.8	60	0.2
Raspberry Fruit Spread					
WEIGHTWATCHERS	153		0.6	39.5	Tr
no added sugar ST DALFOUR	228		0.7	56	0.1
organic MERIDIAN FOODS	128		0.7	31.3	Tr
Raspberry Jam					
Best HARTLEY'S	244		0.5	60.4	0.1
Best, seedless HARTLEY'S	244		0.5	60.4	0.1
reduced sugar STREAMLINE	189		0.5	45.6	0.5
reduced sugar, seedless STREAMLINE	210		0.5	48	0.5
Raspberry Preserve, Scottish					
MACKAYS	253		0.4	63.2	0
Rhubarb & Ginger Jam					
BAXTERS	263		0.5	65	0.1
Rhubarb & Ginger Preserve					
MACKAYS	248		0.2	61.7	0
Seville Orange Fruit Spread					
organic MERIDIAN FOODS	140		0.3	34.8	Tr
Spiced Ginger Preserve					
MACKAYS	261		0.2	64.8	0
Strawberry Conserve					
BAXTERS	263		0.4	65	0.1

Food Type	cal per 100g	cal per portion	pro (g)	carb (g)	fat (g)
Strawberry Fruit Spread					
WEIGHTWATCHERS	156		0.7	39.8	0.1
no added sugar ST DALFOUR	227		0.4	56	0.1
organic MERIDIAN FOODS	140		0.4	34.6	Tr
Strawberry Jam					
Best HARTLEY'S	244		0.4	60.6	0
no-bits HARTLEY'S	256		0.3	63.7	0
reduced sugar STREAMLINE	196		0.3	48	0.3
Strawberry & Redcurrant Jam					
reduced sugar STREAMLINE	192		0.4	46.8	0.3
Three Berry Preserve					
MACKAYS	254		0.3	63.2	0
see also: SUGAR & SWEETENERS					
Nut Butters					
Almond Butter					
MERIDIAN FOODS	627		25.3	6.5	55.5
Brazil Butter					
MERIDIAN FOODS	700		16.5	2.9	69.1
Cashew Butter					
MERIDIAN FOODS	584		20.9	16.7	48.2
Chestnut Purée					
MERCHANT GOURMET	133		1.5	27.1	2
Choc & Nut Spread					
organic WHOLE EARTH	576		22	16.6	46.8
Chocolate Nut Spread	549		6.2	60.5	33

Food Type	cal per 100g	cal per portion	pro (g)	carb (g)	fat (g)
Hazel Butter					
MERIDIAN FOODS	681		17.1	5.8	65.6
Hazelnut Chocolate Spread					
organic GREEN & BLACK	561		4.6	53.7	36.4
Nutella					
FERRERO	530		6.8	56.0	31.0
Peanut Butter					
crunchy	606		24	15	50
crunchy SUN-PAT	587		23.6	10.3	50.1
crunchy, organic, no added sugar MERIDIAN FOODS	612		29.6	11.6	46.0
smooth	611		23	15	51
smooth SUNPAT	581		24	10.1	49.4
smooth, organic, no added sugar MERIDIAN FOODS	579		29.6	11.6	46.0
smooth, organic, no added sugar WHOLE EARTH	596		24.6	9.9	50.8
Tahini					
CYPRESSA	680		25	9.7	60
dark MERIDIAN FOODS	612		21.5	0.9	58.0
light MERIDIAN FOODS	612		21.5	0.9	58.0
Tahini Paste	607		18.5	0.9	58.9

Food Type	cal per 100g	cal per portion	pro (g)	carb (g)	fat (g)
Meat & Poultry					
Bacon & Gammon					
Bacon, Rashers, Back					
dry fried	295		24.2	0	22
fat trimmed, grilled	214		25.7	0	12.3
grilled	287		23.2	0	21.6
microwaved	307		24.2	0	23.3
uncooked	215		16.5	0	16.5
uncooked, smoked WALL'S	223		25.4	0.2	13.5
uncooked, unsmoked WALL'S	214		27.5	0.2	11.5
Bacon, Rashers, Middle					
grilled	307		24.8	0	23.1
Bacon, Rashers, Streaky					
fried	335		23.8	0	26.6
grilled	337		23.8	0	26.9
Gammon					
joint, boiled	204		23.3	0	12.3
rashers, grilled	199		27.5	0	9.9
Lardons					
smoked	234		18.4	Tr	17.8
Pancetta					
smoked	432		14.6	0	41.5
Sausages					
Beef Sausages					
grilled	278		13.3	13.1	19.5

Food Type	cal per 100g	cal per portion	pro (g)	carb (g)	fat (g)
Chicken Frankfurters					
HERTA	204		13	7	16
Cumberland Sausages	328		12.5	2	30
grilled WALL'S	241		13.7	10.5	16.2
Frankfurters					
HERTA	281		12	7	25
Hot & Spicy Sausages					
micro WALL'S	295		10.3	9.9	23.3
Hot Dog Sausages					
jumbo MATTESSONS	320		13	0.5	30
Lincolnshire Sausages					
grilled WALL'S	241		13.7	10.5	16.2
Pork Sausages					
fried	308		13.9	9.9	23.9
grilled WALL'S	257		13.9	11.9	17
micro WALL'S	278		11.2	10.7	20.6
thin, grilled WALL'S	124		6.7	5.8	8.2
Premium Sausages					
grilled	292		16.8	6.3	22.4
Saveloy	296		13.8	10.8	22.3
Beef					
Beef, Fore-rib					
roasted	300		29.1	0	20.4
Beef, Mince					
stewed	209		21.8	0	13.5

Food Type	cal per 100g	cal per portion	pro (g)	carb (g)	fat (g)
Beef, Rump Steak					
lean, grilled	177	31	0	5.9
lean, fried	183	30.9	0	6.6
lean & fat, fried	228	28.4	0	12.7
Beef, Silverside					
lean only, boiled	184	30.4	0	6.9
Beef, Stewing Steak,					
lean & fat, stewed	203	29.2	0	9.6
Beef, Topside					
lean only, roasted well-done	202	36.2	0	6.3
lean & fat, roasted	244	32.8	0	12.5
Grillsteaks, grilled	305	22.1	0.5	23.9
Oxtail, stewed	243	30.5	0	13.4
Lamb					
Lamb, Breast					
lean only, roasted	273	26.7	0	18.5
lean & fat, roasted	359	22.4	0	29.9
Lamb, Cutlets					
lean only, grilled	238	28.5	0	13.8
lean & fat, grilled	367	24.5	0	29.9
Lamb, Leg					
whole, lean only, roasted	203	29.7	0	9.4
whole, lean & fat, roasted	240	28.1	0	14.2

Food Type	cal per 100g	cal per portion	pro (g)	carb (g)	fat (g)
Lamb, Loin Chops					
lean only, grilled	213		29.2	0	10.7
lean & fat, grilled	305		26.5	0	22.1
Lamb, Mince					
stewed	208		24.4	0	12.3
Lamb, Shoulder					
lean only, roasted	218		27.2	0	12.1
lean & fat, roasted	298		24.7	0	22.1
Lamb, Stewing					
lean only, stewed	240		26.6	0	14.8
Pork					
Pork Belly					
rasher, lean & fat, grilled	320		27.4	0	23.4
Pork, Leg					
lean only, roasted	182		33	0	5.5
lean & fat, roasted	215		30.9	0	10.2
Pork, Loin Chops					
lean only, grilled	184		31.6	0	6.4
Pork, Steaks					
lean & fat, grilled	198		32.4	0	7.6
Veal					
Veal					
escalope, fried	196		33.7	0	6.8

Food Type	cal per 100g	cal per portion	pro (g)	carb (g)	fat (g)
Chicken					
Chicken, Breast					
in crumbs, fried	242		18	14.8	12.7
meat only, casseroled	160		28.4	0	5.2
meat only, grilled	148		32	0	2.2
meat only, stir fried	161		29.7	0	4.6
Chicken, Drumsticks					
meat & skin, roasted	185		25.8	0	9.1
Chicken, Leg Quarter					
meat & skin, roasted	236		20.9	0	16.9
Chicken, Light & Dark Meat					
roasted	177		27.3	0	7.5
Chicken, Light Meat					
roasted	153		30.2	0	3.6
Chicken, Wing Quarter					
meat & skin, roasted	226		24.8	0	14.1
Turkey					
Turkey, Breast Fillet					
meat only, grilled	155		35	0	1.7
Turkey, Dark Meat					
roasted	177		29.4	0	6.6
Turkey, Light Meat					
roasted	153		33.7	0	2
Turkey, Meat Only					
roasted	166		31.2	0	4.6

Food Type	cal per 100g	cal per portion	pro (g)	carb (g)	fat (g)
Game					
Duck					
meat only, roasted	195		25.3	0	10.4
meat, fat & skin, roasted	423		20	0	38.1
crispy, Chinese style	331		27.9	0.3	24.2
Goose					
meat, fat & skin, roasted	301		27.5	0	21.2
Pheasant					
meat only, roasted	220		27.9	0	12
Rabbit					
meat only, stewed	114		21.2	0	3.2
Venison					
haunch, meat only, roasted	165		35.6	0	2.5
Offal					
Black Pudding					
dry fried	297		10.3	16.6	21.5
Heart					
lamb, roasted	226		25.3	0	13.9
Kidney					
lamb, fried	188		23.7	0	10.3
ox, stewed	138		24.5	0	4.4
pig, stewed	153		24.4	0	6.1
Liver					
calf, fried	176		22.3	Tr	9.6
chicken, fried	169		22.1	Tr	8.9

Meat & Poultry

Food Type	cal per 100g	cal per portion	pro (g)	carb (g)	fat (g)
lamb, fried	237		30.1	Tr	12.9
ox, stewed	198		24.8	3.6	9.5
pig, stewed	189		25.6	3.6	8.1
Tripe					
dressed, raw	33		7.1	0	0.5
White Pudding	450		7	36.3	31.8
Breaded, Battered or Shaped					
Beef Grillsteaks					
BIRDS EYE	311		15.8	3.6	25.9
ROSS	316		13.3	6	26.6
Beefburgers					
fried	329		28.5	0.1	23.9
grilled	326		26.5	0.1	24.4
BIRDS EYE	274		14.2	2.6	23
100% beef quarter pounder					
BIRDS EYE	292		17.2	0.2	24.7
Angus BIRDS EYE	337		15.8	2.4	29.4
Big Bite BIRDS EYE	262		13.1	6	20.6
Chicken Bites					
BIRDS EYE	206		16.1	8.6	11.9
Chicken Burgers					
Cajun BIRDS EYE	153		21.5	5.8	4.9
quarter pounder BIRDS EYE	253		13.6	16.1	14.9

Food Type	cal per 100g	cal per portion	pro (g)	carb (g)	fat (g)
Chicken Chargrills					
BIRDS EYE	159		17.4	3.1	8.5
Peri Peri BIRDS EYE	159		17.3	5.1	7.7
Chicken Dippers					
breadcrumbs BIRDS EYE	235		13.9	21.3	10.5
crispy BIRDS EYE	239		13.2	16.4	13.4
Chicken Escalope					
ham & cheese BERNARD MATTHEWS	235		11.3	16.3	13.8
Chicken Fillets					
in crispy batter BIRDS EYE	200		21.1	14.7	6.3
Chicken Goujons					
in breadcrumbs BIRDS EYE	275		14.5	19.6	15.4
Chicken Griddlers, BBQ					
BIRDS EYE	159		15.8	5.7	8.1
Chicken Griddlers, Mini					
BIRDS EYE	159		15.8	5.7	8.1
Chicken Kiev					
frozen	294		13	11	22
low fat	207		13	14	11
garlic & herb BIRDS EYE	197		14.5	11	10.5
Chicken Nuggets	281		13	28	13
Cracked Pepper Chicken					
BIRDS EYE	166		17.4	4.4	8.7
Crispy Chicken					
in crispy batter BIRDS EYE	268		13.7	18.5	15.5

Food Type	cal per 100g	cal per portion	pro (g)	carb (g)	fat (g)
Honey & Mustard Seasoned Chicken					
BIRDS EYE	159		17.4	5	7.7
Hot & Spicy Chicken					
in breadcrumbs BIRDS EYE	233		15.1	15.3	12.4
Lamb Burgers					
with rosemary & mint BIRDS EYE	235		17.2	0.6	18.2
Lamb Grillsteaks					
uncooked DALEPAK	286		13.8	5.9	23
uncooked ROSS	300		13.2	3.6	25.4
Meatballs					
BIRDS EYE	302		13.3	5.6	1.7
Mini Kievs					
turkey BERNARD MATTHEWS	183		15.6	8.9	9.4
Southern Fried Chicken					
in breadcrumbs BIRDS EYE	239		14.6	14.2	13.8
Southern Fried Chicken Dippers					
BIRDS EYE	247		14	24.5	10.3
Southern Fried Crispy Chicken					
BERNARD MATTHEWS	183		15.9	7.7	9.8
Thai Seasoned Chicken					
BIRDS EYE	166		17.3	4.5	8.8
Turkey Escalope					
BERNARD MATTHEWS	266		11	20.5	15.6

Food Type	cal per 100g	cal per portion	pro (g)	carb (g)	fat (g)
with creamy pepper sauce					
BERNARD MATTHEWS	241		8.7	17.8	15
Deli & Cold Meat					
Chicken					
breast meat, slices BERNARD					
MATTHEWS	115		19	3	3
roasted, sliced WEIGHTWATCHERS	101		20.7	1.2	1.5
Corned Beef					
PRINCES	223		24.8	0.5	13.5
lean PRINCES	194		25	1	10
Ham					
cooked, wafer thin	84		16.5	Tr	2
cooked, sliced WEIGHTWATCHERS	103		21.5	1	1.4
honey roast	103		20.9	1.9	1.3
honey roast, wafer thin	92		15.8	2	2.3
mustard	117		22	1	2.8
on the bone	136		21	0.8	6
Parma	252		27.8	0.4	15.5
smoked, wafer thin	98		18.5	1	2.2
Wiltshire, sliced	127		24	Tr	3.4
Yorkshire, sliced	151		21.2	Tr	7.3
Haslet	144		13	19	2
Liver Pâté	348		12.6	0.8	32.7
reduced fat	191		18	3	12
Liver Sausage	226		13.4	6	16.7

Food Type	cal per 100g	cal per portion	pro (g)	carb (g)	fat (g)
Luncheon Meat, Canned	279		12.9	3.6	23.8
Pâté, Brussels	345		12	4	31
see also: SAVOURY SPREADS & PASTES					
Peperami					
BBQ PEPERAMI	500		24	2	44
hot PEPERAMI	504		24.5	2.5	44
minis PEPERAMI	536		22	1.7	49
Pork Salami Sausage PEPERAMI	504		24	2.5	44
Polony	281		9.4	14.2	21.1
Pork					
luncheon meat	267		14	3.3	22
oven-baked	183		26	1.4	8
roast with stuffing	160		18	3.3	8
Pork Sausage					
hot & spicy, smoked MATTESSONS	245		14	4.3	19
reduced fat, smoked MATTESSONS	255		14	7	19
smoked MATTESSONS	320		13	0.5	30
Salami	438		20.9	0.5	39.2
German, sliced	309		20	1	25
Milano, sliced	438		23.1	0.3	38.3
Polish kabanos, sliced	366		23	0.1	30.4
Spanish chorizo, sliced	325		22	3	25
Scotch Eggs	241		12	13.1	16
Spam					
tinned HORMEL	289		14.5	3.2	24.2

Food Type	cal per 100g	cal per portion	pro (g)	carb (g)	fat (g)
tinned, light HORMEL	227		16.3	2.1	17
Tongue, Lunch	175		19.5	0.3	10.4
Turkey					
breast, roasted, sliced	115		25	0.6	1.4
breast, sliced BERNARD MATTHEWS	96		19.7	1.6	1.2
Turkey Ham					
honey roast, wafer thin					
BERNARD MATTHEWS	113		16.5	2.5	4.1
wafer thin BERNARD MATTHEWS	103		13.6	3	4.1
Turkey Rashers					
smoked MATTESSONS	99		19.7	1.6	1.6
unsmoked MATTESSONS	99		19.7	1.6	1.6
Meat-free Alternatives					
Chicken Style Burgers					
LINDA MCCARTNEY FOODS	231		11.2	16.1	13.5
Falafel					
as made GRANOSE		149	3.6	17.6	7.1
LINDA MCCARTNEY FOODS	189		7.8	15.2	10.8
Quorn					
myco-protein MARLOW FOODS	92		14.1	1.9	3.2
Quorn Bangers					
MARLOW FOODS	116		11.7	6.6	4.8
Quorn Chilli Sizzling Burger					
MARLOW FOODS	206		17	12	10

Food Type	cal per 100g	cal per portion	pro (g)	carb (g)	fat (g)
Quorn Mince					
MARLOW FOODS	94		14.5	4.5	2
Quorn Mini Savoury Eggs					
MARLOW FOODS	248		15	21	11.5
Sausages					
LINDA MCCARTNEY FOODS	202		22.5	8.3	8.8
Sausages, Cumberland					
CAULDRON FOODS	186		9	16	9.5
Sausages, Lincolnshire					
CAULDRON FOODS	181		10.5	12.2	10
Soya Mince					
unflavoured GRANOSE	82		11.8	8.3	0.2
Tofu (Soya Bean Curd)					
steamed	73		8.1	0.7	4.2
steamed, fried	261		23.5	2	17.7
lightly seasoned, organic					
PROVAMEL	193		18	1	13
'mince', organic PROVAMEL	173		17.5	1	11
organic CAULDRON FOODS	105		12.1	0.6	6
organic PROVAMEL	115		12	1	7
Vegetable Fingers					
BIRDS EYE	188		4.5	24.2	8.1
Vegetable Quarter Pounders					
BIRDS EYE	237		4.7	24.5	13.4

Food Type	cal per 100g	cal per portion	pro (g)	carb (g)	fat (g)
Vegetarian Roast					
LINDA MCCARTNEY FOODS	196		19.4	9.4	9
Veggie Burgers					
LINDA MCCARTNEY FOODS	169		22.8	7.7	5.2
Wensleydale Burgers					
as sold CAULDRON FOODS	179		9	11	11

Food Type

	cal per 100g	cal per portion	pro (g)	carb (g)	fat (g)
Nuts & Seeds					
Almonds					
Blanched/Flaked/Ground	630		25.4	6.5	56
Raw, Mixed, Unblanched	594		20	7	54
Whole HOLLAND & BARRETT	630		25.4	6.5	55.8
Whole JULIAN GRAVES	620		21.3	19.7	50.6
Brazils					
Kernel Only	680		14	3.1	68
Whole HOLLAND & BARRETT	632		14.1	3.1	68.2
Whole JULIAN GRAVES	704		14.3	12.3	66.4
Caraway Seeds					
Dried SCHWARTZ	338		9.2	70	2.4
Cashews					
Kernel Only	576		18	18	48
Whole Nuts, Raw HOLLAND & BARRETT	571		17.7	18.2	48.2
Whole Nuts, Raw JULIAN GRAVES	588		18.2	30.2	43.9
Chestnuts					
Kernel Only	170		2	36.6	2.7
Whole MERCHANT GOURMET	160		2.6	34.7	1.2
Fennel Seeds					
Dried SCHWARTZ	431		18.8	44.1	19.9

Food Type	cal per 100g	cal per portion	pro (g)	carb (g)	fat (g)
Goji Berries					
WHITWORTH	283		12.3	57.7	0.3
Sun-Dried *HOLLAND & BARRETT*	292		2.7	67.7	0.4
Hazelnuts					
Kernel Only	668		17	6	64
Raw *JULIAN GRAVES*	673		15	16.7	60.8
Roast *JULIAN GRAVES*	692		15	17.6	62.4
Macadamias					
Salted	748		7.9	4.8	77.6
Raw *JULIAN GRAVES*	769		7.9	13.8	75.8
Mixed Nuts	607		22.9	7.9	54.1
HOLLAND & BARRETT	581		17.5	7.7	53.4
Peanuts					
Plain, Kernel Only	564		25.8	12.5	46
Paleskin *JULIAN GRAVES*	611		25.8	16.1	49.2
Pecans					
Kernel Only	698		11	6	70
JULIAN GRAVES	740		9.2	13.9	72
Pine Nuts					
Kernel Only	688		14	4	68.6
Kernels *JULIAN GRAVES*	722		13.7	13.1	68.4
Pistachios	620		21	8	56
Raw, Kernels *JULIAN GRAVES*	594		20.6	28	44.4

Food Type	cal per 100g	cal per portion	pro (g)	carb (g)	fat (g)
Roasted & Salted HOLLAND & BARRETT	601		17.9	8.2	55.4
Poppy Seeds	556		20.6	19	44
Pumpkin Seeds JULIAN GRAVES	582		24.5	17.8	45.9
Sesame Seeds SCHWARTZ	634		24.5	16.2	52.4
Sunflower Seeds JULIAN GRAVES	612		22.8	18.8	49.6
Walnuts					
Weighed with Shell	295		6.3	1.4	29.4
Halves JULIAN GRAVES	703		15.2	13.7	65.2
Halves HOLLAND & BARRETT	688		14.7	3.3	68.5

Food Type	cal per 100g	cal per portion	pro (g)	carb (g)	fat (g)
Oils & Fats					
Oils					
Crisp 'n' Dry					
SPRY	828		0	0	92
spray SPRY	522		0	0	58
Coconut Oil	899		Tr	0	99.9
Corn Oil					
MAZOLA	829		0	0	92.1
Garlic Infused Oil					
BLUE DRAGON	820		0.1	1	90.6
Grapeseed Oil					
MERIDIAN FOODS	899		0	0	99.9
Olive Oil	899		Tr	0	99.9
BERTOLLI	820		0	0	91
FILIPPO BERIO	822		0	0	91.3
NAPOLINA	823		0	0	91.4
OLIVIO	828		0	0	92
extra virgin, organic					
MERIDIAN FOODS LTD	899		0	0	99.8
spray NAPOLINA	495		0	0	55
spray, light FRY	522		Tr	Tr	55.2
spray, mild & light					
FILIPPO BERIO	822		0	0	91.3
Palm Oil	899		Tr	0	99.9
Peanut Oil	899		Tr	0	99.9

Food Type	cal per 100g	cal per portion	pro (g)	carb (g)	fat (g)
Rapeseed Oil	899		Tr	0	99.9
FARRINGTON'S	817		0.6	1	90.1
Safflower Oil	899		Tr	0	99.9
organic MERIDIAN FOODS LTD	899		0	0	99.8
Sesame Oil	898		0.2	0	99.7
organic MERIDIAN FOODS LTD	899		0	0	99.8
organic, toasted MERIDIAN FOODS LTD	899		0	0	99.8
toasted BLUE DRAGON	828		4.1	32.3	92
Soya Oil	899		Tr	0	99.9
SOYOLA	900		0	0	100
Sunflower Oil					
FLORA	828		0	0	92
organic MERIDIAN FOODS LTD	899		0	0	99.8
spray FLORA	522		0	0	58
spray, light FRY	522		Tr	Tr	55.2
spray, light, butter flavour FRY	522		Tr	Tr	55.2
Vegetable Oil	899		Tr	0	99.9
Vegetable & Olive Oil Blend					
OLIVIO	828		0	0	92
Wheatgerm Oil	899		Tr	0	99.9
Fats					
Cooking Fat					
COOKEEN	900		0	0	100

Food Type	cal per 100g	cal per portion	pro (g)	carb (g)	fat (g)
Crisp 'n' Dry					
solid SPRY	900		0	0	100
Dripping					
beef	891		Tr	Tr	99
Ghee					
butter	898		Tr	Tr	99.8
palm	897		Tr	Tr	99.7
vegetable	895		Tr	Tr	99.4
Lard	891		Tr	0	99
Suet, Shredded	826		Tr	12.1	86.7
ATORA	830		0.9	10.1	87.4
light ATORA	695		2.7	31	62.2
White Flora					
FLORA	855		0	0	95

see also: **BUTTER & MARGARINES**

Oils & Fats

Food Type

	cal per 100g	cal per portion	pro (g)	carb (g)	fat (g)
Pasta, Rice & Noodles					
see also: SNACK MEALS					
Pasta					
Dry Lasagne Sheets					
egg NAPOLINA	362		13	70	3.3
verdi	350		13	68	2.9
Dry Pasta, All Shapes					
standard NAPOLINA	362		12	77	0.7
wholewheat NAPOLINA	335		14	63	3
Dry Pasta, Tortiglioni					
semi wholewheat, organic					
SEEDS OF CHANGE	348		11.5	72	1.5
Dry Pasta, Trotolle					
verdi organic SEEDS OF CHANGE	348		11.5	72	1.5
Fresh Egg Pasta					
conchiglie, fusilli, penne	147		6.3	26.9	1.6
lasagne sheets	169		6.3	31.8	1.8
spaghetti	148		5.3	28.2	1.5
tagliatelle	141		5.1	26.2	1.7
Gnocchi					
Italian	153		3.9	34.1	0.1
Macaroni					
as sold MARSHALLS	348		12.5	69.9	2
Pasta, Brocolli & Green Beans					
frozen, Steam Fresh BIRDS EYE	76		3.1	13.7	1

Food Type	cal per 100g	cal per portion	pro (g)	carb (g)	fat (g)
Pasta, Peas & Sweetcorn					
frozen, Steam Fresh BIRDS EYE	135		4.2	22.3	3.2
Pre-Cooked Pasta, All Shapes					
Express Pasta DOLMIO	136		5.3	26.3	1.1
My Dolmio DOLMIO	140		5.9	26	1.4
Rice & Millet Pasta					
ORGRAN	351		7	77.4	1.6
Spaghetti					
as sold NAPOLINA	362		12	77	0.7
Stuffed Fresh Pasta					
meat ravioli	251		11.8	29	9.8
cheese, tomato & basil ravioli	224		9.2	31.6	6.7
chicken & mushroom tortellini	287		9.8	40.2	9.7
four cheese tortellini	197		8	30	5
garlic & herb tortellini	217		6.9	31.7	7
ham & cheese tortellini	170		6	23	6
spinach & ricotta cannelloni	206		8.1	13.9	13.1
Dry Rice					
Arborio Risotto Rice					
as sold	349		7	78.5	0.8
organic RISO GALLO	349		7	78	1
Bahia Paella Rice					
as sold	345		6.6	78.3	0.6
Basmati Rice					
TILDA	348		8.6	77.6	0.4

Food Type	cal per 100g	cal per portion	pro (g)	carb (g)	fat (g)
Basmati & Wild Rice					
TILDA	349		9.4	77	0.4
Beef Savoury Rice					
BATCHELORS	359		8.9	75.7	2.3
Brown Basmati Rice					
TILDA	347		9.2	71.4	2.7
Camargue Red Rice					
as sold MERCHANT GOURMET	343		7	72.6	2.7
Carnaroli Rice					
as sold RISO GALLO	349		7	78	1
Cheese, Onion & Wine Risotto					
as prepared, per sachet (140g)					
AINSLEY HARRIOTT		650	9.7	111.3	18
Chicken Savoury Rice					
BATCHELORS	346		9.6	73.1	1.7
as prepared, per sachet (120g)					
AINSLEY HARRIOTT		201	5.4	41.8	1.3
Chinese Savoury Rice					
BATCHELORS	359		9.4	75.5	2.2
Egg Fried Rice					
BATCHELORS	369		8.6	77.9	2.6
Garlic Butter Savoury Rice					
BATCHELORS	370		8.6	78.7	2.3

Gem Calorie Counter

Food Type	cal per 100g	cal per portion	pro (g)	carb (g)	fat (g)
Golden Savoury Rice					
BATCHELORS	357		8.7	76.5	1.8
Golden Vegetable Savoury Rice					
as prepared, per sachet (120g)					
AINSLEY HARRIOTT		199	5	42.6	0.9
Long Grain Rice					
UNCLE BEN'S	344		7.3	76	1.3
Mediterranean Style Tomato & Pepper Risotto					
as prepared, per sachet (140g)					
AINSLEY HARRIOTT		599	9.7	102.5	16.6
Mild Curry Savoury Rice					
BATCHELORS	355		8	76.1	2.1
Mixed Vegetable Savoury Rice					
as prepared, per sachet (120g)					
AINSLEY HARRIOTT		201	5.1	43	0.9
Mushroom Savoury Rice					
BATCHELORS	356		10.7	73.6	2.1
Mushroom & Pepper Savoury Rice					
as prepared, per sachet (120g)					
AINSLEY HARRIOTT		196	5.9	40.4	1.2
Pudding Rice	345		6.6	78.3	0.6
Sushi Rice					
BLUE DRAGON	343		7.2	77.5	0.5

Food Type	cal per 100g	cal per portion	pro (g)	carb (g)	fat (g)
Thai Jasmine Rice					
TILDA	348		7.1	79.5	0.2
Valencia Paella Rice	348		6.3	78.9	0.8
Wholegrain Rice					
UNCLE BEN'S	344		8	73	2.2
Wild Mushroom Risotto					
as prepared, per sachet (140g)					
AINSLEY HARRIOTT		596	11.1	99.2	17
Pre-cooked Rice					
Bacon & Mushroom Risotto					
UNCLE BEN'S	179		4.3	30.2	4.6
Basmati Rice					
Boil in the Bag UNCLE BEN'S	148		3.2	30	1.7
Express UNCLE BEN'S	148		3.2	30	1.7
microwave (300g) AINSLEY HARRIOTT		216	4.7	44.7	2
wok UNCLE BEN'S	165		3.5	32.8	2.2
Basmati & Thai					
Boil in the Bag UNCLE BEN'S	177		3.4	35.8	2.3
Brown Steamed Basmati Rice					
TILDA	136		3.6	25.7	2.1
Chicken & Mushroom Risotto					
UNCLE BEN'S	180		4.9	32.3	3.5
Chinese Style Express Rice					
UNCLE BEN'S	156		3.4	30.7	2.2

Food Type	cal per 100g	cal per portion	pro (g)	carb (g)	fat (g)
Egg Fried Express Rice					
UNCLE BEN'S	173		4	29.9	4.2
Egg Fried Steamed Basmati Rice					
TILDA	115		2.7	19.4	2.9
Garlic & Coriander Flavoured Rice					
Express UNCLE BEN'S	156		3.2	31.4	1.9
Garlic & Herb Wok Rice					
UNCLE BEN'S	172		3.4	34.1	2.5
Golden Vegetable Express Rice					
UNCLE BEN'S	148		3.3	29.7	1.8
Lemon & Rosemary Express Rice					
UNCLE BEN'S	156		3.2	31.2	2
Lime & Coriander Steamed Basmati Rice					
TILDA	126		2.6	24.5	2
Long Grain Rice					
Boil in the Bag UNCLE BEN'S	344		7.3	76	1.3
Express UNCLE BEN'S	146		3	31.1	1
microwave (300g) AINSLEY					
HARRIOTT		210	3.8	44.3	2
Long Grain & Wild Rice					
Express UNCLE BEN'S	342		8.5	75	1
Mexican Express Rice					
UNCLE BEN'S	157		3.2	35	1.8

Food Type	cal per 100g	cal per portion	pro (g)	carb (g)	fat (g)
Mushroom Express Rice					
UNCLE BEN'S	157		3.2	31.7	1.9
Mushroom Steamed Basmati Rice					
TILDA	119		2.6	20.9	2.8
Oriental Wok Rice					
UNCLE BEN'S	163		3.3	32	2.5
Original Vegetable Rice, frozen					
BIRDS EYE	100		4	20.2	0.3
Pilau Express Rice					
UNCLE BEN'S	164		3.2	30.8	3.1
Pilau Steamed Basmati Rice					
TILDA	120		2.6	22.1	2.3
Savoury Chicken Express Rice					
UNCLE BEN'S	148		3.5	29	1.9
Special Fried Express Rice					
UNCLE BEN'S	163		4.3	27.4	4.1
Spicy Mexican Express Rice					
UNCLE BEN'S	165		3.8	30.3	3.2
Sun Dried Tomato & Mascarpone Risotto					
NEW COVENT GARDEN	111		3.3	16.3	3..6
Sweet & Spicy Express Rice					
UNCLE BEN'S	169		2.7	30.5	4

Food Type	cal per 100g	cal per portion	pro (g)	carb (g)	fat (g)
Thai Curry Express Rice					
UNCLE BEN'S	154		3.2	30.2	2.3
Thai Sticky Rice					
microwave (300g) AINSLEY HARRIOTT		213	3.5	45.2	2
Thai Sweet Chilli Express Rice					
UNCLE BEN'S	346		7.9	78	0.4
Tomato & Basil Express Rice					
UNCLE BEN'S	181		3.5	32.2	4.2
Tomato & Italian Herbs Risotto					
UNCLE BEN'S	187		3.5	31.4	5.2
Vegetable Pilau Express Rice					
UNCLE BEN'S	156		3	29	3.1
Wholegrain Rice					
Boil in the Bag UNCLE BEN'S	344		8	73	2.2
Express UNCLE BEN'S	346		7.9	78	0.4
Wholegrain Rice with Mediterranean Vegetables					
Express UNCLE BEN'S	172		3.8	27.2	5.3
Wild Mushroom & Parmesan Risotto					
NEW COVENT GARDEN	88		2.4	13.7	2.6
Wok Rice					
Basmati UNCLE BEN'S	165		3.5	32.8	2.2
garlic & herbs UNCLE BEN'S	172		3.4	34.1	2.5
Oriental UNCLE BEN'S	163		3.3	32	2.5

Food Type	cal per 100g	cal per portion	pro (g)	carb (g)	fat (g)
Noodles, Dry					
Crispy Noodles					
BLUE DRAGON	350		2.4	84	0.5
Egg Noodle Nests					
fine BLUE DRAGON	356		13.8	70	1.7
medium BLUE DRAGON	356		13.8	70	1.7
Egg Noodles					
fine SHARWOOD	217		7.5	43.8	1.3
medium SHARWOOD	217		7.5	43.8	1.3
organic BLUE DRAGON	345		12	70	1.9
Rice Noodles					
SHARWOOD	382		6.5	86.8	1
fine BLUE DRAGON	349		1	86.1	0.3
medium BLUE DRAGON	349		1	86.1	0.3
Stir Fry Noodles					
SHARWOOD	170		5.4	32.5	2
Noodles, Cooked					
Egg Noodles					
boiled	62		2.2	13	0.5
Pad Thai Ribbon Noodles					
SHARWOOD	164		5.5	30	2.4
Quick Wok Noodles					
chilli infused BLUE DRAGON	191		6.1	33.6	0.7
coriander infused BLUE DRAGON	173		6.2	33.7	0.8
medium wheat BLUE DRAGON	193		5.9	34	1

Food Type	cal per 100g	cal per portion	pro (g)	carb (g)	fat (g)
medium wholewheat BLUE DRAGON	157		4.6	28.6	0.4
wide wheat BLUE DRAGON	190		6	33.4	0.6
Straight to Wok Noodles					
Singapore AMOY	116		1.6	27.4	0.1
Thread AMOY	155		4.8	28.4	2.8
Udon AMOY	139		4.9	28.8	1.1

Food Type	cal per 100g	cal per portion	pro (g)	carb (g)	fat (g)
Pizza					
American Hot Pizza					
PIZZA EXPRESS	221		11	27.3	7.6
American Pizza					
PIZZA EXPRESS	221		11.6	27.5	7.2
Bistro Baguette					
Jambon DR OETKER	203		7.3	27.8	6.9
Tomate-Fromage DR OETKER	231		6.1	27.9	10.5
Cajun Chicken Pizza					
Delicia GOODFELLA'S	220		12.9	22.6	8.7
California Cheese Pizza Edge to Edge					
Thin & Crispy CHICAGO TOWN	302		15	23.8	16.3
Cheese & Tomato Pizza					
deep pan base	249		12.4	35.1	7.5
French bread base	230		10.6	31.4	7.8
thin base	277		14.4	33.9	10.3
as prepared MCCAIN	361		12.6	34.8	7.9
Chicken Pesto Pizza					
Solo GOODFELLA'S	257		10.8	26.9	11.8
Four Cheese Stuffed Crust					
Takeaway CHICAGO TOWN	268		12.6	31.8	10
French Bread Pizza					
cheese & tomato FINDUS	240		11	31	7.5
ham & pineapple FINDUS	190		8.5	32	3.5

Food Type	cal per 100g	cal per portion	pro (g)	carb (g)	fat (g)
pepperoni supreme FINDUS	22		8.5	29	7.5
Friday Fever Pizza					
cheese supreme GOODFELLA'S	256		16.2	20	12
chicken fajita GOODFELLA'S	199		11.9	18.5	8.7
Funghi Pizza					
Ristorante DR OETKER	234		7.8	22.9	12.3
Ham & Pineapple Deep Pan					
CHICAGO TOWN	257		9.4	31	10.6
individual CHICAGO TOWN		424	15.5	51	17.5
Hawaii Pizza					
Ristorante DR OETKER	215		8.6	25.6	8.6
Loaded Cheese					
Deeply Delicious GOODFELLA'S	521		25	53.7	22.9
Manhattan Chicken Melt Edge to Edge					
thin & crispy CHICAGO TOWN	237		12.3	23.3	10.5
Margherita Pizza					
PIZZA EXPRESS	206		12.1	28.8	4.8
deep pan SAN MARCO	233		8.3	38.1	6.9
Solo GOODFELLA'S	247		10.7	29	9.8
Meat Combo					
thin dish CHICAGO TOWN	267		10.9	30.4	11.3
Meat Speciale					
Solo GOODFELLA'S	252		10.9	27.3	11

Food Type	cal per 100g	cal per portion	pro (g)	carb (g)	fat (g)
Micro Pizza					
chargrilled chicken, as prepared MCCAIN	287		15.5	33.3	10.2
cheese & tomato, as prepared MCCAIN	319		16	38.5	11.2
pepperoni, as prepared MCCAIN	340		16.6	38.8	13.2
Mozzarella Pizza					
Delicia GOODFELLA'S	266		11.5	25.4	13.1
La Bottega GOODFELLA'S	456		20.9	53.6	20.1
Ristorante DR OETKER	263		10.9	24.1	13.6
New York Deli Edge to Edge					
thin & crispy CHICAGO TOWN	263		12	21.8	14.2
Pepperoni Classico Pizza					
La Bottega GOODFELLA'S	456		20.9	53.6	11.5
Pollo Pizza					
Ristorante DR OETKER	213		8.7	23.6	9.2
Pollo ad Astra Pizza					
PIZZA EXPRESS	190		11.6	25.2	4.7
Pepperoni Pizza					
deep pan CHICAGO TOWN	313		11.3	30	16.4
deep pan SAN MARCO	244		8.2	33.6	8.5
deep pan, individual CHICAGO TOWN		515	18.5	49.5	27
Deeply Delicious GOODFELLA'S	521		25	53.7	22.9
Delicia GOODFELLA'S	396		19.1	33.1	20.8
Solo GOODFELLA'S	267		10.8	26.6	13

Food Type	cal per 100g	cal per portion	pro (g)	carb (g)	fat (g)
Pepperoni Stuffed Crust Pizza					
Takeaway CHICAGO TOWN	283		12.4	31	12.2
Pizza Bases					
light & crispy NAPOLINA	291		7.9	58	3
mini NAPOLINA	291		7.9	58	3
Pizza Topping					
tomato sauce with herbs NAPOLINA	49		0.9	6.3	2.2
Quattro Formaggi Pizza					
PIZZA EXPRESS	243		12.1	26.5	9.8
Ristorante DR OETKER	266		10.8	24.1	14
Sloppy Giuseppe					
PIZZA EXPRESS	186		10.6	23.3	5.6
Speciale Pizza					
Ristorante DR OETKER	251		10.9	23.3	12.6
Spicy Chicken Jolt					
Deeply Delicious GOODFELLA'S	257		13.1	30.9	9
Sweet Chilli Chicken Pizza					
La Bottega GOODFELLA'S	379		19.2	50.6	14.3
Three Cheese & Tomato Pizza					
WEIGHTWATCHERS	156		9.8	25.6	1.6
Tuna Melt Pizza					
Solo GOODFELLA'S	250		11.5	281	10.2
Vegetale Piccante					
Ristorante DR OETKER	203		7.3	24.3	8.4

Pizza

Food Type

	cal per 100g	cal per portion	pro (g)	carb (g)	fat (g)
Quiches, Pies & Savoury Pastries					
Chicken Curry Pie					
canned FRAY BENTOS	158		7.8	13.3	8.2
Chicken Lattice					
bacon & cheddar cheese					
BIRDS EYE	293		13.4	21	17.3
cheddar cheese & broccoli					
BIRDS EYE	288		12.6	22.7	16.3
Chicken Pie					
each BIRDS EYE		455	12	39	28
Chicken Slice, Spicy					
each GINSTER'S		449	12	38.5	27.4
Chicken, Ham & Mushroom Pie					
frozen MCDOUGALL'S	261		9	18	17
Chicken & Asparagus Pie					
frozen MCDOUGALL'S	231		9.4	20.5	12.4
Chicken & Leek Deep-Filled Pie					
frozen MCDOUGALL'S	227		8.6	21.5	11.8
Chicken & Mozzarella Bake					
each GINSTER'S		478	17.2	39	28.2
Chicken & Mushroom Pie					
individual		423	11.4	36.5	25.7
canned FRAY BENTOS	167		7.4	12.1	9.9
canned PRINCE'S	194		9.9	18	9.1

Food Type	cal per 100g	cal per portion	pro (g)	carb (g)	fat (g)
Chicken & Mushroom Slice					
each GINSTER'S		465	13.5	32.8	31.1
Cheese, Leek & Red Onion Plaits					
LINDA MCCARTNEY FOODS	278		6.7	25.9	16.5
Cheese & Onion Pie					
individual		325	7	27	21
Cheese & Onion Slice					
each GINSTER'S		306	8.7	24.5	19.3
Cornish Pastie	267		6.7	25	16.3
Cornish Pasty					
each GINSTER'S		549	12.1	52.7	32.2
large, each GINSTER'S		626	13	42.3	45
Country Pies					
LINDA MCCARTNEY FOODS	248		5.1	26.1	13.7
Game Pie	381		12.2	34.7	22.5
Ham & Cheese Slice					
each GINSTER'S		512	15.3	36.8	33.7
Ham & Mozzarella Bake					
each GINSTER'S		426	13	25.3	30.4
Hot Pockets Crispy Pastries					
bacon & egg, each MAGGI		392	13.4	34	22.5
Bolognese, each MAGGI		375	10.8	34.3	21.6
ham & egg, each MAGGI		349	11.1	33.8	18.8
Melton Mowbray Pork Pie					
DICKINSON & MORRIS	387		11.5	22.9	27.7

Food Type	cal per 100g	cal per portion	pro (g)	carb (g)	fat (g)
each GINSTER'S		497	14.8	32.9	34.1
mini, each DICKINSON & MORRIS		199	5.6	12.4	14.1
Minced Beef & Onion Pie	241		7	24	13
canned FRAY BENTOS	178		5.6	14.3	10.9
frozen, each BIRDS EYE		470	10	42	29
Minced Beef & Potato Lattice	378		9.4	29.1	24.9
Peppered Steak Pie					
frozen MCDOUGALL'S	307		8.1	23.2	20.2
Peppered Steak Slice					
each GINSTER'S		513	17.1	29	36.5
Ploughman's Roll					
each GINSTER'S		543	12.6	34.3	39.4
Pork Pie					
mini, each GINSTER'S		177	6	10.6	12.2
Quiche Lorraine	246		6.6	18.5	16.2
WEIGHTWATCHERS	177		8.7	17.5	8
Quiche					
bacon, leek & cheese					
WEIGHTWATCHERS	186		7.4	21	8.1
cheese & egg recipe	315		12.4	17.1	22.3
three cheese & spring onion	237		9	12	17
Sausage Roll					
flaky pastry	383		9.9	25.4	27.6
large, each GINSTER'S		545	13.4	39.8	36.9

Food Type	cal per 100g	cal per portion	pro (g)	carb (g)	fat (g)
Sausage Rolls					
LINDA MCCARTNEY FOODS	278		13.1	26	13.7
Sausage & Onion Plait	376		9.9	18.6	29.1
Steak Pie					
individual		298	9	25	18
Steak Slice					
each GINSTER'S		406	13.9	31.3	25.1
Steak & Ale Pie					
canned FRAY BENTOS	164	7.8	13	8.6	11.7
Steak & Gravy Pie					
frozen MCDOUGALL'S	224		9.8	21.9	10.8
Steak & Kidney Pie					
individual		298	8	26	18
pastry top only	286		15.2	15.9	18.4
classic, canned FRAY BENTOS	154		8.1	11.4	8.4
frozen, each BIRDS EYE		460	13	37	29
Steak & Kidney Pudding					
canned FRAY BENTOS	213		8	19.1	11.6
Steak & Mushroom Pie					
canned FRAY BENTOS	182		6.7	13.2	11.3
frozen MCDOUGALL'S	239		6.7	21.6	14
Steak with Three Veg Pie					
canned FRAY BENTOS	179		5.6	14.2	11.1
Vegetable & Cheese Pie	289		4.7	29.7	16.8

Quiches, Pies & Savoury Pastries

Food Type	cal per 100g	cal per portion	pro (g)	carb (g)	fat (g)
Yorkshire Pudding					
frozen	262		8	35	10
frozen AUNT BESSIE'S	291		10.5	36.6	11.3
Yorkshire Pudding Batters					
frozen AUNT BESSIE'S	276		9.1	32.6	10.8

see also: READY MEALS; FISH &
SEAFOOD

Food Type	cal per 100g	cal per portion	pro (g)	carb (g)	fat (g)

Ready Meals

see also: QUICHES, PIES & SAVOURY
PASTRIES; FISH & SEAFOOD

Traditional

Food Type	cal per 100g	cal per portion	pro (g)	carb (g)	fat (g)
Beef Hotpot					
Healthy Options BIRDS EYE	96		5.5	12.6	2.6
WEIGHTWATCHERS	66		3.6	8.1	2.1
Beef Stew					
canned SHIPPAMS	92		10.6	6.4	1.4
Beef Stew & Dumplings					
BIRDS EYE	89		4.7	9.9	3.4
Taste of Home HEINZ	78		3.2	9.4	3.1
Cauliflower Cheese					
BIRDS EYE	93		4.8	6	5.5
Chicken Casserole & Dumplings					
WEIGHTWATCHERS	83		6.8	9.5	2
Chicken Curry					
canned SHIPPAMS	88		11.1	3.4	3.3
Chicken Hotpot					
WEIGHTWATCHERS	82		4.7	10.4	2.3
Chicken in a Creamy Mushroom Sauce					
WEIGHTWATCHERS	103		7	12.4	2.8
Chicken Kiev					
frozen	294		13	11	22

Food Type	cal per 100g	cal per portion	pro (g)	carb (g)	fat (g)
low fat	207		13	14	11
garlic & herb BIRDS EYE	197		14.5	11	10.5
Chicken Supreme					
canned SHIPPAMS	116		11.8	3.4	6.1
with rice BIRDS EYE	125		6.6	18.8	2.6
Chicken with Vegetables					
ST DALFOUR	89		7.2	9.8	2.3
Chicken & Vegetable Casserole					
taste of home HEINZ	74		3.5	6.7	3.7
Cottage Pie					
WEIGHTWATCHERS	72		5.5	8.5	1.7
healthy options BIRDS EYE	83		4.9	11.9	1.8
Country Vegetable Casserole					
taste of home HEINZ	74		3.5	6.7	3.7
Crispy Pancakes					
minced beef FINDUS	160		6.5	25	3.5
three cheeses FINDUS	190		7	25	6.5
Faggots in a Rich West Country Sauce					
MR BRAIN'S	125		6.5	11.3	6
Lancashire Lamb Hotpot					
Taste of Home HEINZ	65		2.9	8.8	2
Macaroni Cheese					
BIRDS EYE	155		5.5	22.1	4.9
WEIGHTWATCHERS	81		4.7	12.4	1.3

Food Type	cal per 100g	cal per portion	pro (g)	carb (g)	fat (g)
canned BRANSTON	95		3.2	13.9	2.9
canned HEINZ	85		3.7	11	2.9
frozen FINDUS	150		5.5	16	7
per pot AINSLEY HARRIOTT		467	14.5	66.8	16
Minced Beef with Onions in Gravy					
PRINCES	95		11.5	6.7	2.5
Roast Beef Dinner					
BIRDS EYE	90		7.3	10.3	2
in gravy BIRDS EYE	78		13.4	2.2	1.7
Roast Chicken Dinner					
BIRDS EYE	103		9.5	9.6	2.9
in gravy BIRDS EYE	66		12.6	1.8	0.9
Roast Lamb Dinner					
BIRDS EYE	107		5.8	12	4
Roast Pork Dinner					
BIRDS EYE	100		6.5	11.2	3.2
Roast Turkey Dinner					
BIRDS EYE	93		6.5	11.5	2.3
Sausages in Cider Gravy with Vegetable Mash					
WEIGHTWATCHERS	78		4.7	11	1.7
Shepherd's Pie					
BIRDS EYE	85		4.5	11.5	2.3
WEIGHTWATCHERS	67		3.2	9.3	2

Food Type	cal per 100g	cal per portion	pro (g)	carb (g)	fat (g)
Steak & Kidney in a Rich Gravy					
PRINCES	123		15.5	4	5
Stewed Steak with Gravy					
PRINCES	128		16.8	4	5
Spam Fritters					
HORMEL	276		10.2	18.1	18.1
Tender Steak in Creamy Peppercorn & Onion Sauce					
WEIGHTWATCHERS	109		5	12.9	4.2
Toad in the Hole					
AUNT BESSIE'S	238		13.1	20.6	11.4
Vegetarian Roast					
LINDA MCCARTNEY FOODS	196		19.4	9.4	9
Chinese					
Beef & Blackbean with Rice					
WEIGHTWATCHERS	90		5	14.6	1.3
Chicken Chow Mein	80		7	8.4	2
Chow Mein with Noodles					
VESTA	135		5.4	23.1	2.3
Spring Rolls					
as prepared	224		3.7	32	9
Sweet & Sour Chicken					
Healthy Options BIRDS EYE	112		4.8	20.7	1.1

Food Type	cal per 100g	cal per portion	pro (g)	carb (g)	fat (g)
Italian					
Bolognese Bake					
WEIGHTWATCHERS	81		6.1	9.6	2
Creamy Vegetable Pasta					
per pot AINSLEY HARRIOTT		414	10.8	70	10.1
Lasagne					
frozen, cooked	143		7.4	15.7	6.1
beef BIRDS EYE	121		6.9	15	3.7
beef, Pasta Preso FINDUS	100		5.5	12	3.5
beef WEIGHTWATCHERS	86		5.3	10	2.8
vegetarian LINDA MCCARTNEY FOODS	125		6.3	12.4	5.6
Mediterranean Vegetable Pasta					
WEIGHTWATCHERS	69		2.1	14.8	0.1
Risotto	233		3.5	35.1	9.7
chicken & lemon WEIGHTWATCHERS	95		5.9	12.5	2.3
Spaghetti Bolognese					
BIRDS EYE	107		6	15	2.6
WEIGHTWATCHERS	97		5.6	14	2.1
Spicy Three Bean Bakes					
LINDA MCCARTNEY FOODS	232		4.5	23.2	13.5
Spicy Tomato Pasta					
per pot AINSLEY HARRIOTT		369	10.2	77.2	2.1
Tomato & Basil Chicken with Potato Wedges					
WEIGHTWATCHERS	75		4.7	9.2	2.1

Food Type	cal per 100g	cal per portion	pro (g)	carb (g)	fat (g)

see also: **PASTA, RICE & NOODLES**

Indian

Beef Curry

canned SHIPPAM'S — 129 — 12.7 — 5.7 — 6.2

Beef Curry with Rice

BIRDS EYE — 114 — 5.7 — 15.8 — 3.1

VESTA — 109 — 3.6 — 18.5 — 2.3

Chicken Curry

healthy options BIRDS EYE — 99 — 5.3 — 17.3 — 1

Chicken Curry with Rice

BIRDS EYE — 100 — 6.5 — 14.6 — 2

WEIGHTWATCHERS — 92 — 5.2 — 14.6 — 1.4

Chicken Tikka Masala with Rice

BIRDS EYE — 117 — 5.3 — 17.7 — 2.8

WEIGHTWATCHERS — 91 — 6.1 — 11.9 — 2.1

Indian Daal Curry Veg Pot

each INNOCENT — — 323 — 15.6 — 41.7 — 10.3

Prawn Curry with Rice

BIRDS EYE — 113 — 3.3 — 15.8 — 4.1

Samosas

meat — 272 — 11.4 — 18.9 — 17.3

vegetable — 223 — 4 — 23.5 — 12.5

Mexican

Burrito Dinner Kit

salsa OLD EL PASO — 43 — 1.6 — 9.1 — 0.5

Food Type	cal per 100g	cal per portion	pro (g)	carb (g)	fat (g)
spice mix OLD EL PASO	276		11	50	0.5
tortilla OLD EL PASO	344		8.7	51.1	11.7
Chicken Fajita Wraps					
FINDUS	150		5.5	22	4.5
Chilli Beef Wraps					
FINDUS	180		7	25	6.5
Chilli non Carne					
LINDA MCCARTNEY FOODS	73		5.6	8.1	2
Crispy Chicken Fajita Dinner Kit					
salsa OLD EL PASO	42		1.6	9	0.5
seasoning mix OLD EL PASO	327		11	65	2.7
tortilla OLD EL PASO	344		8.7	51.1	11.7
Enchilada Dinner Kit					
spice mix OLD EL PASO	264		7.4	46	4.6
tom sauce OLD EL PASO	56		2	12	0.5
tortilla OLD EL PASO	3115		10	44	11
Roasted Tomato & Pepper					
Fajita Dinner Kit					
salsa OLD EL PASO	37		1.3	8	0.5
spice mix OLD EL PASO	271		8.2	52.1	2.8
tortilla OLD EL PASO	323		8.3	51.9	8.9
Smokey BBQ Fajita Dinner Kit					
salsa OLD EL PASO	43		1.6	9.1	0.5
spice mix OLD EL PASO	285		7.9	56	1.8
tortilla OLD EL PASO	344		8.7	51.1	11.7

Food Type	cal per 100g	cal per portion	pro (g)	carb (g)	fat (g)
Spicy Chilli & Wedges					
Healthy Options BIRDS EYE	74		4.7	9.7	1.8
Taco Dinner Kit					
salsa OLD EL PASO	43		1.6	9.1	0.5
spice mix OLD EL PASO	298		4.6	60	2.6
taco shells OLD EL PASO	506		7	61	26
World					
Beef Stroganoff	165		9.4	16.2	6.7
Doner Kebabs					
SNACKSTERS	245		8.7	28.6	10.6
Moroccan Squash Tagine Veg Pot					
each INNOCENT		296	12.4	40.8	9.2
Moussaka manufacturer	124		6	10.2	6.6
Pea & Broccoli Rice Veg Pot					
each INNOCENT		303	15.5	38.8	9.5
Thai Coconut Curry Veg Pot					
each INNOCENT		288	12.6	35	10.7
Tuscan Bean Stew Veg Pot					
each INNOCENT		281	13.2	36.9	9

see also: **SNACK MEALS**

Food Type	cal per 100g	cal per portion	pro (g)	carb (g)	fat (g)
Savoury Spreads & Pastes					
Anchovy Paste					
ADMIRAL	150		21.9	1.8	5.3
SHIPPAMS	125		13.8	4.6	5.5
Ardennes Pâté	320		13	3.8	28
Beef Paste	194		17	0.1	14
PRINCES	180		15.7	2.8	11.9
Beef Spread					
SHIPPAMS	205		850	16.9	13.4
Bloater Paste					
SHIPPAMS	144		13.8	3	8.5
Brussels Pâté	403		10.7	2.2	39
Chicken Paste	184		16	0.8	13
Chicken Sandwich Filler					
HEINZ	199		4.1	12.4	14.8
Chicken Spread					
SHIPPAMS	185		16.9	11.7	18.6
Chicken & Ham Paste					
PRINCES	169		16.2	3.2	10.1
Chicken & Stuffing Paste					
PRINCES	143		15.2	0.1	9.1
Crab Pâté, Orkney					
luxury CASTLE MACLELLAN	221		7.3	5.5	18.9
Crab Spread					
SHIPPAMS	165		13.2	5	10.2
Fish Paste	170		15.3	3.7	10.5

Food Type	cal per 100g	cal per portion	pro (g)	carb (g)	fat (g)
Herbs & Garlic Yeast Pâté					
TARTEX	230		7	10	18
Mackerel Pâté, peppered					
JOHN WEST	297		15.7	Tr	26
Marmite Yeast Extract					
MARMITE	252		38.7	24.1	0.1
Pâté					
mushroom CAULDRON FOODS	119		2.8	4.3	10.1
mushroom GRANOVITA	229		9.6	10.6	16.5
olive GRANOVITA	3.8		8.3	6.6	27.6
vegetable GRANOVITA	227		7.2	7.9	18.5
Ready Spready					
organic GRANOVITA	222		10	5	18
garlic & herb, organic GRANOVITA	159		7	8	11
herb, organic GRANOVITA	234		12	6	18
mushroom, organic GRANOVITA	235		11	5	19
Salmon Pâté					
JOHN WEST	272		14.9	Tr	23.5
Salmon Spread					
SHIPPAMS	185		12	7.6	12.1
Sandwich Spread					
HEINZ	225		1	24.9	13.1
light HEINZ	161		1.1	18.2	9.2
Sardine & Tomato Paste					
PRINCES	125		15.6	2.8	5.8
Spam Spreaders					
HORMEL	175		14.5	2	11.7

Food Type	cal per 100g	cal per portion	pro (g)	carb (g)	fat (g)
bacon HORMEL	175		14.5	2	11.7
black pepper HORMEL	175		14.5	2	11.7
onion & chive HORMEL	175		14.5	2	11.7
Sweet Tomato, Lentil & Basil Pâté					
CAULDRON FOODS	154		7.5	15.6	6.8
Tartex Yeast Pâté					
original TARTEX	239		7	10	19
Tasty & Tender Chicken					
Coronation PRINCES	138		15.8	6.9	5.2
sweetcorn & light mayonnaise					
PRINCES	153		18.5	5.2	6.5
tikka PRINCES	135		19.6	3.8	4.6
Toast Toppers					
chicken & mushroom HEINZ	56		5.1	5.7	1.4
ham & cheese HEINZ	95		7.3	7.3	4.1
mushroom & bacon HEINZ	94		6.9	6.6	4.4
Tuna Pâté					
JOHN WEST	263		15.3	Tr	22.4
Tuna & Mayonnaise Paste					
PRINCES	208		15.2	5	14.2
Tuna & Sweetcorn Sandwich Filler					
HEINZ	185		5.9	13.1	12.1
Vegemite					
KRAFT	191		25.6	19.5	0.9

Food Type	cal per 100g	cal per portion	pro (g)	carb (g)	fat (g)
Snack Meals					
Bacon Supernoodles					
BATCHELORS	175		3.2	23.1	7.8
Barbecue Beef Supernoodles					
BATCHELORS	173		3.1	22.5	7.8
Beef Noodle Lunchbox					
each BLUE DRAGON		418	7.2	50.5	19.9
Beef & Black Pepper Noodle Town					
BLUE DRAGON	458		8.3	59.8	20.6
Beef & Black Pepper Snack Noodles					
BLUE DRAGON	454		9	60.4	19.6
Beef & Tomato Pot Noodle					
as prepared POT NOODLE COMPANY		424	10.8	62.2	14.7
king pot, as prepared POT NOODLE COMPANY		528	13.2	76	19
Bombay Bad Boy Pot Noodle					
as prepared POT NOODLE COMPANY		415	10.6	59	15.2
king pot, as prepared POT NOODLE COMPANY		543	13.9	77.5	19.7
Brunchettas					
ploughman's relish GOLDEN VALE	271		12.3	23.3	14.6
red pepper & onion relish GOLDEN VALE	274		12.7	19.1	16.5

Food Type	cal per 100g	cal per portion	pro (g)	carb (g)	fat (g)
Cheese & Ham Micro Toastie					
as prepared MCCAIN		457	21.4	56.7	16
Chicken Chow Mein					
Supernoodles To Go					
each BATCHELORS		377	8.5	51.2	15.3
Chicken Noodle Lunchbox					
each BLUE DRAGON		418	7.2	50.5	19.9
Chichen Satay Pot Noodle					
as prepared POT NOODLE COMPANY		413	9.2	60.8	14.9
Chicken Supernoodles					
BATCHELORS	174		3.1	22.8	7.8
Chicken Supernoodles To Go					
each BATCHELORS		389	9	53.4	15.5
Chicken & Chilli Noodle Town					
BLUE DRAGON	467		9.3	60.7	20.8
Chicken & Herb Supernoodles					
98% fat-free BATCHELORS	112		3.7	23.3	0.4
Chicken & Mushroom Pot Noodle					
as prepared POT NOODLE COMPANY		418	10.4	60.7	14.8
king pot, as prepared					
POT NOODLE COMPANY	545	13.9	78.9	19.3	
Chicken & Spring Onion Snack					
Noodles					
BLUE DRAGON	448		9.2	61	18.6

Food Type	cal per 100g	cal per portion	pro (g)	carb (g)	fat (g)
Chicken & Vegetable Curry Pot					
big eat, each HEINZ		393	18.9	38.3	18.3
Chinese Chow Mein Pot Noodle					
as prepared POT NOODLE COMPANY		416	10.2	60.8	6.9
Chinese Spare Rib					
Supernoodles To Go					
each BATCHELORS		396	8	53.8	16.6
Chow Mein Noodle Town					
BLUE DRAGON	464		9.3	20.8	14.8
Crispy Duck Noodle Town					
BLUE DRAGON	452		8.3	59.4	20.2
Curry Supernoodles To Go					
each BATCHELORS		403	8.4	54.8	16.7
Dairylea Lunchables					
chicken, each KRAFT		265	16.5	22.5	11.5
ham, each KRAFT		285	16.5	23	13
Fridge Raiders Chicken Bites					
chicken tikka MATTESSONS	181		19.9	2	10.4
chinese spare rib MATTESSONS	178		20.4	3.9	9
roast chicken MATTESSONS	193		20.7	3.5	11.3
southern fried chicken					
MATTESSONS	174		20.1	3.3	8.9
sweet chilli MATTESSONS	179		20.1	3.5	9.4
Hot & Sour Cup Noodle					
as prepared TIGER TIGER		390	6	60	14

Food Type	cal per 100g	cal per portion	pro (g)	carb (g)	fat (g)
Lamb Hot Pot Pot Noodle					
as prepared POT NOODLE COMPANY		448	10.1	68.8	14.7
Mild Mexican Chilli Supernoodles					
as served BATCHELORS	175		3.1	23.2	7.8
Mug Shot Chicken Noodle Snack					
each SYMINGTON'S		214	5.7	44.3	1.5
Mug Shot Creamy Cheese Pasta Snack					
each SYMINGTON'S		301	10	51.8	6
Mug Shot Sweet 'n' Sour Noodle Snack					
each SYMINGTON'S		239	6.1	53.6	1.9
Mug Shot Tomato 'n' Herb Pasta Snack					
each SYMINGTON'S		265	5.9	55.7	2.1
Mushroom Noodle Town					
BLUE DRAGON	466		9.3	60.3	20.8
Oriental Chicken Noodle Wok					
BLUE DRAGON	370		7.7	51	15
Original Curry Pot Noodle					
each POT NOODLE COMPANY		431	10	64	15
king pot, *as prepared* POT NOODLE COMPANY		561	12.6	83.8	19.5

Food Type	cal per 100g	cal per portion	pro (g)	carb (g)	fat (g)
Ravioli in Tomato Sauce					
HEINZ	77		2.4	13	1.7
cheese & tomato HEINZ	82		2.4	13.4	2
mini vegetable HEINZ	72		2.2	12.2	1.6
Roast Chicken Supernoodles To Go					
each BATCHELORS		389	9	53.4	15.5
Southern Fried Chicken Pot Noodle					
as prepared POT NOODLE COMPANY		427	10	63.3	14.9
Southern Fried Chicken Supernoodles					
BATCHELORS	175		3.2	22.8	7.9
Spaghetti Bolognese					
HEINZ	79		3.4	13.2	1.5
Spaghetti Bolognese Pot					
big eat, each HEINZ		278	17.4	41	4.9
Spaghetti Hoops					
HEINZ	53		1.6	11.1	0.3
snap pots HEINZ	59		1.6	12.7	0.3
Spaghetti Hoops 'n' Hotdogs in a Smoky Bacon Sauce					
HEINZ	81		3	10.1	3.2
Spaghetti in Tomato Sauce					
HEINZ	61		1.7	13	0.2

Food Type	cal per 100g	cal per portion	pro (g)	carb (g)	fat (g)
multigrain HEINZ	60		1.7	12.7	0.3
WEIGHTWATCHERS	49		1.8	9.9	0.2
with parsley WEIGHTWATCHERS	49		1.8	9.7	0.3
Spaghetti with Sausages in Tomato Sauce					
HEINZ	89		3.4	11.1	3.5
Spicy Thai Noodle Wok					
BLUE DRAGON	371		7.2	52	14.9
Sweet Chilli Chicken Noodle Wok					
BLUE DRAGON	400		7	45	11
Sweet Thai Chilli Supernoodles					
98% fat-free BATCHELORS	113		3.6	23.7	0.4
Sweet & Spicy Pot Noodle					
as prepared POT NOODLE COMPANY		423	9.8	62.3	15
Thai Curry Cup Noodle					
per pack TIGER TIGER		407	8.4	62.2	13.9
Thai Spice Cup Noodle					
per pack TIGER TIGER		413	7	58	17
Tikka Masala Pot Noodle					
as prepared POT NOODLE COMPANY		428	11.4	61.5	15.2
Tom Yum Cup Noodle					
per pack TIGER TIGER		411	7	62	15
Won Ton Noodle Town					
BLUE DRAGON	465		9.1	60	20.9

Food Type	cal per 100g	cal per portion	pro (g)	carb (g)	fat (g)
WOT? Not in a Pot Noodle					
beef & tomato POT NOODLE COMPANY	81		1.6	10.5	3.6
chicken & mushroom POT NOODLE COMPANY	81		1.6	10.5	3.6
southern fried chicken POT NOODLE COMPANY	81		1.4	10.8	3.7
sweet & sour POT NOODLE COMPANY	82		1.2	11.1	3.6

Food Type	cal per 100g	cal per portion	pro (g)	carb (g)	fat (g)
Soups					
Asparagus Cup Soup					
low calorie, per sachet AINSLEY					
HARRIOTT		36	0.5	6.4	0.9
Autumn Three Bean & Tomato Soup					
Farmers' Market HEINZ	44		2.3	7.5	0.5
Autumn Vegetable Soup					
Healthy Choice BAXTERS	46		1.9	9	0.3
Autumn Vegetable & Lentil Soup					
HEINZ	46		2.3	8.6	0.3
Bacon, Leek & Potato Soup					
Big Soup HEINZ	54		1.9	6.6	2.1
Bean Fusion Soup					
LOYD GROSSMAN	79		3.4	10.1	2.7
Beef Broth					
HEINZ	45		2.2	7.5	0.7
Big Soup Heinz	43		2.2	6.9	0.7
Beef Consommé					
BAXTERS	13		2.6	0.7	Tr
Beef, Mushroom & Red Wine Soup					
Farmers' Market HEINZ	51		2.4	6.4	1.8

Food Type	cal per 100g	cal per portion	pro (g)	carb (g)	fat (g)
Beef & Tomato Soup					
Cup-A-Soup, per sachet					
BATCHELORS		83	1.4	15.8	1.6
Beef & Vegetable Soup					
Big Soup Heinz	48		2.9	7.2	0.8
Soupfulls, each BATCHELORS		180	13.6	25.2	2.8
Beef & Winter Vegetable Soup					
BAXTERS	47		2.3	6.9	1.1
Broccoli, Stilton & Bacon Soup					
BAXTERS	75		2.5	5.4	4.8
Broccoli & Cauliflower Soup					
Slim-A-Soup Special, per					
sachet BATCHELORS		59	1	9.5	1.9
Broccoli & Stilton Soup					
NEW COVENT GARDEN	56		2.9	2.7	3.7
as sold KNORR	519		11.2	30.8	39
Butternut Squash & Red Pepper Soup					
BAXTERS	39		0.7	6.9	1
Cajun Spicy Vegetable Soup					
Slim-A-Soup Special, per					
sachet BATCHELORS		52	1.7	9.4	0.8
Carrot, Bean & Quinoa Soup, Chunky					
Healthy Choice BAXTERS	48		2	8.6	0.6

Food Type	cal per 100g	cal per portion	pro (g)	carb (g)	fat (g)
Carrot, Onion & Chick Pea Soup					
Healthy Choice BAXTERS	41		1.9	8	0.2
Carrot & Butter Bean Soup					
BAXTERS	55		1.7	7.7	1.9
Carrot & Coriander Soup					
BAXTERS	40		0.8	6.1	1.4
LOYD GROSSMAN	51		0.6	6.4	2.5
NEW COVENT GARDEN	43		0.6	5.2	2.2
as sold KNORR	394		6.9	50.1	18.2
Cup Soup, per sachet AINSLEY HARRIOTT		98	1.2	19.1	1.9
organic SEEDS OF CHANGE	37		0.6	4.7	1.8
Carrot & Lentil Soup					
WEIGHTWATCHERS	29		1.3	5.7	0.1
Chicken Broth					
BAXTERS	31		1.4	5.6	0.3
Chicken Consommé					
BAXTERS	8		1.1	0.9	Tr
Chicken Noodle Soup					
HEINZ	31		1.2	6	0.3
as sold KNORR	328		14.9	56.7	4.6
clear WEIGHTWATCHERS	17		0.8	3.1	0.2
Cup-A-Soup Special, per sachet BATCHELORS		96	4.3	17	1.2

Food Type	cal per 100g	cal per portion	pro (g)	carb (g)	fat (g)
Chicken Noodle with Sweetcorn Soup					
BAXTERS	34		1.4	5.8	0.6
Chicken Noodle & Vegetable Soup					
Slim-A-Soup, per sachet					
BATCHELORS		55	1.6	10	1
Chicken, Potato & Bacon Soup					
Big Soup HEINZ	54		3.1	6.2	1.9
Chicken, Potato & Leek Soup					
WEIGHTWATCHERS	34		1.2	5.3	0.9
Chicken Soup					
NEW COVENT GARDEN	94		3.7	6.6	5.9
WEIGHTWATCHERS	30		1.2	4	1
Cup-A-Soup, per sachet					
BATCHELORS		83	1.1	8.3	5
Chicken & Country Vegetable Soup					
Farmers' Market HEINZ	72		3.5	6	3.7
Soupfulls, each BATCHELORS		184	12.4	23.2	4.4
Chicken & Herb Soup					
Farmers' Market HEINZ	61		2.2	7.8	2.3
Chicken & Leek Soup					
big soup HEINZ	63		3	8.2	2

Food Type	cal per 100g	cal per portion	pro (g)	carb (g)	fat (g)
Cup-A-Soup, per sachet					
BATCHELORS		96	1.2	12.2	4.7
Cup Soup, per sachet AINSLEY					
HARRIOTT		105	1.3	17.2	3.4
Chicken & Mushroom					
Slim-A-Soup, per sachet					
BATCHELORS	60		1.3	9	2.1
Soupfulls, each BATCHELORS		246	12.4	22	12
Chicken & Sweetcorn Soup					
BAXTERS	36		1.4	6	0.7
BLUE DRAGON	33		1.6	4.5	0.9
Chinese, Soups of the world					
HEINZ	45		1.9	6.2	1.4
Slim-A-Soup, per sachet					
BATCHELORS		58	1.3	9.1	1.8
Chicken & Vegetable Casserole					
Soup, Chunky					
Healthy Choice BAXTERS	47		2.4	7.8	0.7
Chicken & Vegetable Soup					
HEINZ	33		1.2	6.2	0.4
LOYD GROSSMAN	68		0.5	8	3.8
Big Soup HEINZ	47		2.9	7.4	0.6
Cup-A-Soup, per sachet BATCHELORS	143		1.7	19	6.7
Cup Soup, per sachet AINSLEY					
HARRIOTT		99	1.2	15.7	3.4

Food Type	cal per 100g	cal per portion	pro (g)	carb (g)	fat (g)
Healthy Choice BAXTERS	39		1.9	6.8	0.5
Soupfulls, each BATCHELORS		182	12.4	23.2	4.4
Chilli Beef with Lentils & Buckwheat Soup					
BAXTERS	57		3.7	9.3	0.5
Chilli Beef & Bean Soup					
chunky, Healthy Choice BAXTERS	58		3.8	9	0.7
mexican, Soups of the World HEINZ	70		4.5	9	1.8
Chinese Chicken Noodle					
Cup-A-Soup Extra, per sachet BATCHELORS		101	3.5	19.1	1.2
Cock-a-Leekie Soup					
BAXTERS	23		1	3.7	0.5
Country Garden Soup					
BAXTERS	33		1	6	0.5
Country Vegetable Soup					
WEIGHTWATCHERS	31		1.1	6.1	0.2
chunky, Healthy Choice BAXTERS	46		2	8.8	0.3
Country Vegetable & Herb Soup					
Farmers' Market HEINZ	38		1.2	5.7	1.2
Cream of Asparagus Soup					
BAXTERS	65		1.1	5.8	4.2
Cup-A-Soup with croutons, per sachet BATCHELORS		134	0.7	18	6.6

Food Type	cal per 100g	cal per portion	pro (g)	carb (g)	fat (g)
Cream of Celery Soup					
condensed BATCHELORS	46		0.6	3	3.5
Cream of Chicken Soup					
BAXTERS	70		2.1	5.4	4.4
HEINZ	52		1.7	4.7	3
condensed BATCHELORS	100		2.1	7.8	6.7
Cream of Chicken & Mushroom Soup					
HEINZ	52		1.7	4.7	3
Cream of Chicken & Vegetable Casserole					
Cup-A-Soup, per sachet					
BATCHELORS		52	0.5	6.9	2.5
Cream of Leek Soup					
BAXTERS	57		1.1	3.8	4.2
Cream of Mushroom Soup					
BAXTERS	61		1	5.6	3.8
HEINZ	52		1.6	5.2	2.8
condensed BATCHELORS	109		1.3	6.7	8.6
Cup-A-Soup with croutons, per sachet BATCHELORS		121	0.9	15.2	6.3
Cream of Red Pepper Soup					
BAXTERS	52		0.9	5.9	2.8
Cream of Tomato Soup					
BAXTERS	62		1	8.4	2.7

Food Type	cal per 100g	cal per portion	pro (g)	carb (g)	fat (g)
HEINZ	57		0.9	6.6	3
condensed BATCHELORS	154		1.7	21.9	6.6
organic HEINZ	55		1	7	2.6
Cream of Tomato & Basil Soup					
HEINZ	57		0.9	6.6	3
Cream of Vegetable Soup					
Cup-A-Soup, per sachet					
BATCHELORS		135	1.8	17.3	6.5
Creamy Asparagus Soup					
Cup Soup, per sachet AINSLEY					
HARRIOTT		108	1.4	14.6	5
Creamy Broccoli & Cauliflower Soup					
Cup-A-Soup, per sachet					
BATCHELORS		107	1.6	13.7	5.1
Creamy Carrot & Coriander Soup					
Cup-A-Soup, per sachet					
BATCHELORS		93	1.4	16.4	2.4
Creamy Chicken Soup					
Cup Soup, per sachet AINSLEY					
HARRIOTT		105	1.3	17.2	3.4
Creamy Chicken & Mushroom Soup					
BAXTERS	52		1.7	5.3	2.7

Food Type	cal per 100g	cal per portion	pro (g)	carb (g)	fat (g)
Crofters' Thick Vegetable Soup					
as sold KNORR	353		10.2	54.7	10.2
Cullen Skink Soup					
BAXTERS	85		5.7	7.7	3.5
Flame Roasted Red Pepper & Tomato Soup					
BAXTERS	59		0.9	6.8	3.1
Florida Spring Vegetable Soup					
as sold KNORR	277		10	43.3	6.8
French Onion Soup					
BAXTERS	29		0.9	6.1	0.1
as sold KNORR	317		11.5	52.3	6.3
Cup Soup, per sachet AINSLEY HARRIOTT		87	1.6	17.3	1.3
Golden Vegetable Soup					
Cup-A-Soup, per sachet BATCHELORS		83	1.1	14.3	2.4
Harvest Vegetable Soup					
Soupfulls, each BATCHELORS		160	5.6	33.6	Tr
Hearty Leek & Potato Soup					
Cup Soup, per sachet AINSLEY HARRIOTT		97	0.9	17.8	2.5
Hearty Vegetable Broth					
WEIGHTWATCHERS	43		2	8.2	0.2

Food Type	cal per 100g	cal per portion	pro (g)	carb (g)	fat (g)
Highlander's Broth					
BAXTERS	47		1.8	6.5	1.5
Hot & Sour Soup					
Cup Soup, per sachet AINSLEY HARRIOTT		53	1.2	11.8	1
Indian Mild Chicken Curry Soup					
Soups of the World HEINZ	74		3.6	5.9	4.1
Italian Bean & Pasta Soup					
Healthy Choice BAXTERS	51		2.1	10.1	0.2
Italian Chicken, Tomato & Red Pepper Soup					
HEINZ	50		1.6	4.6	2.8
Italian Minestrone Soup					
Soups of the World HEINZ	73		2	12.2	1.8
Italian Tomato with Basil Soup					
BAXTERS	48		2.1	7.9	0.9
Italian Wedding Soup					
BAXTERS	48		2.1	6.9	1.3
Lamb & Vegetable Soup					
Big Soup HEINZ	60		3	9.1	1.3
Leek, Potato & Pea					
Cup Soup, low calorie, per sachet AINSLEY HARRIOTT		73	2.6	14	0.7
Leek & Chicken Soup					
as sold KNORR	440		10.6	36	28.1

Food Type	cal per 100g	cal per portion	pro (g)	carb (g)	fat (g)
Leek & Potato Soup					
NEW COVENT GARDEN	50		1.2	6.8	2
Cup-A-Soup Extra, per sachet					
BATCHELORS		137	2.7	19.5	5.3
Lentil Soup					
HEINZ	42		2.3	7.7	0.2
spicy, organic SEEDS OF					
CHANGE	71		2.8	9.8	2.2
Lentil & Bacon Soup					
BAXTERS	52		3.2	7.7	0.9
Lentil & Smoked Bacon Soup					
NEW COVENT GARDEN	77		4.7	10.3	1.9
Lentil & Vegetable Soup					
Healthy Choice BAXTERS	42		2.3	7.8	0.2
Lobster Bisque					
BAXTERS	44		2.7	3.8	2
Mediterranean Tomato Soup					
BAXTERS	31		0.9	6.3	0.2
Cup Soup, per sachet AINSLEY					
HARRIOTT		87	1.4	15.6	2.1
Slim-A-Soup, per sachet					
BATCHELORS		55	0.9	9.8	1.3
Mediterranean Tomato &					
Lentil Soup					
WEIGHTWATCHERS	46		2.3	7.8	0.6

Soups

Food Type	cal per 100g	cal per portion	pro (g)	carb (g)	fat (g)
Minestrone Soup					
BAXTERS	34		1.5	5.9	0.5
HEINZ	42		1	5.8	1.6
NEW COVENT GARDEN	37		1.4	5.8	0.9
as sold KNORR	306		11	53.8	4.7
Chunky, Big Soup HEINZ	41		1.6	6.6	0.9
Cup-A-Soup Special, per sachet BATCHELORS		90	1.6	17	1.7
hearty, Farmers' Market HEINZ	41		1.4	6.9	0.9
organic SEEDS OF CHANGE	65		1.4	7.4	3.3
Slim-A-Soup with croutons, per sachet BATCHELORS		55	1.3	10.2	1
Tuscan WEIGHTWATCHERS	44		1.1	7.3	1.1
with wholemeal pasta, Healthy Choice BAXTERS	34		0.9	7	0.2
Minted Lamb Hotpot Soup					
Big Soup HEINZ	58		2.9	8.6	1.3
Miso					
instant, sachet, each SANCHI		27	1.3	4.5	0.3
white, instant, sachet, each CLEARSPRING		35	2.4	3.9	1.1
Moroccan Lamb, Chick Pea & Cous Cous Soup					
Soups of the World HEINZ	61		3	8.9	1.5

Food Type	cal per 100g	cal per portion	pro (g)	carb (g)	fat (g)
Moroccan Tomato & Chickpea Soup					
WEIGHTWATCHERS	31		1.3	5.9	0.3
Mulligatawny Beef Curry Soup					
HEINZ	52		2	7.1	1.8
Mushroom Potage					
BAXTERS	78		1.5	6.6	5.1
LOYD GROSSMAN	59		0.9	5.5	3.8
Mushroom Soup					
WEIGHTWATCHERS	28		1.1	4.5	0.7
Cup Soup, low calorie, per sachet AINSLEY HARRIOTT		80	2.8	14	1.4
Mushroom & Croutons Soup					
Cup Soup HEINZ	40		0.7	4.5	2.1
Oxtail Soup					
BAXTERS	48		1.8	7.4	1.2
HEINZ	39		1.9	6.7	0.5
Cup-A-Soup, per sachet					
BATCHELORS		83	2.2	11.2	3.3
Pea & Ham Soup					
BAXTERS	60		3.5	8.3	1.4
HEINZ	54		2.7	9	0.7
NEW COVENT GARDEN	58		3.6	7.4	1.6
Pea & Smoked Ham Soup					
Farmers' Market HEINZ	40		3.5	5.6	0.4

Food Type	cal per 100g	cal per portion	pro (g)	carb (g)	fat (g)
Plum Tomato & Mascarpone Soup					
NEW COVENT GARDEN	52		1.3	5.3	2.8
Potato, Leek & Thyme Soup					
Farmers' Market HEINZ	57		0.9	6.6	3
Potato & Leek Soup					
BAXTERS	44		1.2	8.1	0.8
HEINZ	46		0.8	6.6	1.8
Puy Lentil & Tomato Soup					
Healthy Choice BAXTERS	57		3.1	10.5	0.3
Red Lentil & Vegetable Soup					
BAXTERS	40		2.2	7.4	0.2
Rich Tomato & Basil Soup Cup-A-Soup, per sachet					
BATCHELORS		97	1.3	17.3	2.5
Rich Woodland Mushroom Soup Cup-A-Soup, per sachet					
BATCHELORS		110	1.3	15	5
Roast Tomato & Parmesan Soup					
BAXTERS	44		1.2	5.6	1.9
Root Vegetable & Butternut Squash Soup					
BAXTERS	45		1.9	8.7	0.3

Food Type	cal per 100g	cal per portion	pro (g)	carb (g)	fat (g)
Royal Game Soup					
BAXTERS	36		2.2	6	0.3
Sausage & Vegetable Soup					
Big Soup HEINZ	46		2.3	7.5	0.8
Scotch Broth					
BAXTERS	48		2	7.8	1
HEINZ	42		1.5	6	1.3
Scotch Vegetable Soup					
BAXTERS	43		2	7.6	0.5
Seafood Chowder					
BAXTERS	75		3	5.8	4.4
Shropshire Pea Soup					
Cup Soup, per sachet AINSLEY					
HARRIOTT		92	2	16.6	1.9
Slow Cooked Lamb with Root					
Vegetable Soup					
Farmers' Market HEINZ	56		2.5	6.6	2.2
Smoked Bacon & Three Bean					
Soup, Chunky					
Healthy Choice BAXTERS	58		2.9	8.8	1.2
Smoked Haddock Chowder					
NEW COVENT GARDEN	59		2.3	8.3	1.8
Smokey Bacon, Leek & Potato					
Soup					
Big Soup HEINZ	54		1.9	6.6	2.1

Soups

Food Type	cal per 100g	cal per portion	pro (g)	carb (g)	fat (g)
Soup Bowls					
butternut squash, carrot & red pepper BAXTERS	38		0.7	6.5	1
medley of country vegetables BAXTERS	46		1.9	8.9	0.3
smoked bacon & mixed bean BAXTERS	47		2.4	8.4	0.4
spicy lentil, tomato & vegetable BAXTERS	50		2.2	8.9	0.6
tomato & sweet basil BAXTERS	48		2.1	7.9	0.9
Spiced Lentil & Potato Soup					
WEIGHTWATCHERS	40		2	7.7	0.2
Spicy Lentil Soup					
Cup Soup, per sachet AINSLEY HARRIOTT		86	2.4	16.4	1.2
Cup Soup, low calorie, per sachet AINSLEY HARRIOTT		67	2.7	13.3	0.3
organic SEEDS OF CHANGE	71		2.8	9.8	2.2
Slim-A-Soup, per sachet BATCHELORS		64	2	13.4	0.3
Spicy Lentil & Vegetable Soup, Chunky					
Healthy Choice BAXTERS	50		2.3	8.9	0.6

Food Type	cal per 100g	cal per portion	pro (g)	carb (g)	fat (g)
Spicy Mixed Bean Soup					
Big Soup HEINZ	39		2.3	6.7	0.3
Spicy Parsnip Soup					
BAXTERS	52		1.2	6.1	2.5
NEW COVENT GARDEN	39		0.9	5.8	1.3
Spicy Tomato & Rice with Sweetcorn Soup					
Healthy Choice BAXTERS	51		1.9	10.2	0.3
Spring Vegetable Soup					
HEINZ	34		0.8	6.8	0.4
Steak & Potato Soup					
Big Soup HEINZ	50		3	7.7	0.8
Tangy Tomato & Rice Soup					
WEIGHTWATCHERS	39	1.1	8.4	0.1	0.2
Thai Green Curry Soup					
BLUE DRAGON	89		0.8	8.6	5.7
Soups of the World HEINZ	71		2.1	6.5	4.1
Thai Red Curry Soup					
BLUE DRAGON	97		0.9	11.8	5.1
Three Bean Soup					
organic SEEDS OF CHANGE	59		2.1	9.7	1.3
Three Bean & Smoked Bacon Soup					
Farmers' Market HEINZ	66		4	7.5	2.2

Food Type	cal per 100g	cal per portion	pro (g)	carb (g)	fat (g)
Tomato Soup					
WEIGHTWATCHERS	25		0.7	4.5	0.5
Cup Soup, low calorie, per					
sachet AINSLEY HARRIOTT		70	1.9	14.5	0.5
Cup-A-Soup, per sachet					
BATCHELORS		92	0.7	17.2	2.3
Tomato, Basil & Crème Fraîche					
Soup					
organic SEEDS OF CHANGE	68		1.2	12	1.7
Tomato, Sweet Chilli &					
Pasta Soup					
HEINZ	37		0.8	8	0.1
Tomato & Basil Soup					
LOYD GROSSMAN	46		0.8	6.4	1.9
Tomato & Brown Lentil Soup					
Healthy Choice BAXTERS	48		2.6	9	0.2
Tomato & Butter Bean Soup					
BAXTERS	40		1.2	6.1	1.2
Tomato & Chunky Vegetable					
Soup					
NEW COVENT GARDEN	47		1.6	6.7	1.5
Tomato & Herb Soup					
Cup Soup HEINZ	25		0.5	4.5	0.6
Cup Soup, per sachet AINSLEY					
HARRIOTT		79	1.4	16.2	1

Food Type	cal per 100g	cal per portion	pro (g)	carb (g)	fat (g)
Tomato & Pasta Soup					
Soupfulls, each BATCHELORS		208	7.2	33.2	5.2
Tomato & Red Pepper with					
Herb Soup					
Farmers' Market HEINZ	39		1.3	5.2	1.4
Tomato & Sweet Basil Soup					
NEW COVENT GARDEN	44		1.3	5.2	2
Tomato & Vegetable Soup					
Cup-A-Soup Special, per					
sachet BATCHELORS	108		2.8	18.4	2.6
Vegetable Chowder					
Cup Soup, per sachet AINSLEY					
HARRIOTT		83	1.4	13	2.8
Vegetable Soup					
HEINZ	45		1.1	8.2	0.8
Cup Soup HEINZ	25		0.4	4.7	0.5
Cup Soup, low calorie, per					
sachet AINSLEY HARRIOTT		74	1.9	15	0.7
Vegetable Soup, Chunky					
Big Soup HEINZ	52		1.7	9.2	0.9
Wild Mushroom Soup					
NEW COVENT GARDEN	38		1.2	4.8	1.6
Cup Soup, per sachet AINSLEY					
HARRIOTT		84	0.9	12.3	3.5
Farmers' Market HEINZ	31		0.9	4.4	1.1

Food Type	cal per 100g	cal per portion	pro (g)	carb (g)	fat (g)
Wiltshire Cured Ham & Golden Sweetcorn Soup					
BAXTERS	69		2.4	8.1	3
Winter Vegetable Soup					
BAXTERS	40		1.5	8.1	0.2
HEINZ	34		0.8	7.3	0.2
Wonton Soup					
BLUE DRAGON	25		1.2	2	1.3
Woodland Mushroom Soup					
Farmers' Market HEINZ	44		0.9	4.7	2.4

Food Type	cal per 100g	cal per portion	pro (g)	carb (g)	fat (g)
Sugar & Sweeteners					
see also: JAMS, MARMALADES					
& SWEET SPREADS					
Amber Sugar Crystals					
TATE & LYLE	398		0	100	0
Barley Malt Extract					
organic MERIDIAN FOODS	316		4	76	Tr
Date Syrup					
MERIDIAN FOODS	292		1.2	72	0.1
Golden Syrup	298		0.3	79	0
TATE & LYLE	325		0.5	80.5	0
Icing Sugar					
TATE & LYLE	398		0	99.5	0
golden, unrefined cane BILLINGTON'S	398		0.8	98.1	0.2
Jaggery	367		0.5	97.2	0
Maple Syrup					
Canadian, amber	253		Tr	63	0.1
Canadian CLARK'S	265		0.1	63	0.1
Canadian ROWSE	265		Tr	63	0.1
organic MERIDIAN FOODS	334		Tr	85.3	0.3
Molasses					
blackstrap, organic					
MERIDIAN FOODS	268		2	65	Tr
Sucron					
SILVER SPOON	371		0	98.9	0

Food Type	cal per 100g	cal per portion	pro (g)	carb (g)	fat (g)
Sugar					
caster TATE & LYLE	400		0	100	0
cube, white TATE & LYLE	400		0	100	0
dark brown, soft SILVER SPOON	395		0.4	97.3	0.5
dark brown, soft TATE & LYLE	378		Tr	94.5	0
dark muscovado, unrefined cane BILLLINGTON'S	370		Tr	92.5	0
demerara, cane TATE & LYLE	396		0	98.5	0
demerara, unrefined cane BILLLINGTON'S	396		Tr	99	0
fruit TATE & LYLE	400		0	100	0
golden granulated, unrefined cane BILLLINGTON'S	398		Tr	99.6	0
granulated TATE & LYLE	400		0	100	0
granulated, light SILVER SPOON	400		0	100	0
jam SILVER SPOON	398		0.2	98.6	0.3
jam TATE & LYLE	397		0	100	0
light brown, soft SILVER SPOON	397		0.4	98.4	0.2
light brown, soft TATE & LYLE	384		Tr	95.5	0
light muscovado, unrefined cane BILLLINGTON'S	384		Tr	96	0
Sweetness & Light					
SILVER SPOON	374		1.4	92.2	0
Treacle					
black	257		1.2	67.2	0
black LYLE'S	290		1.7	64	0

Food Type	cal per 100g	cal per portion	pro (g)	carb (g)	fat (g)
Sweets & Chocolate					
Aero					
bubbles NESTLÉ	526		6.3	20.4	30.5
milk chocolate NESTLÉ	531		6.3	17.5	30.9
mint NESTLÉ	546		6.5	20.4	31
After Dinner Mint Leaves					
organic GREEN & BLACK	575		6.4	37.3	44.4
After Eight Mints					
bitesize NESTLÉ	432		3.8	36.9	16.4
chocolate mint straws NESTLÉ	526		5.1	2.5	31
dark chocolate NESTLÉ	461		5	4.2	12.9
Animal Mix					
BASSETT	315		3	75.8	Tr
Aniseed Imperials					
per pack BASSETT	170		0.2	42.1	0.2
Aquadrops					
MARS	247		0.1	94.5	1
Blue Riband					
NESTLÉ	513		4.8	46.6	25.3
Boiled Sweets	327		Tr	87.1	Tr
Bonbons					
fruit BASSETT	375		Tr	93.6	Tr
lemon BASSETT	425		Tr	83.7	9.8
strawberry BASSETT	380		Tr	75.7	8.7
toffee BASSETT	420		Tr	83.7	9.3

Food Type	cal per 100g	cal per portion	pro (g)	carb (g)	fat (g)
Boost					
glucose, each CADBURY		315	3.4	35.1	17.8
Bounty					
MARS	469		3.7	63.8	23.9
Bournville					
CADBURY	495		4	61.1	26.3
99 calories, each CADBURY		95	1.4	4.9	7.8
coffee CADBURY	535		7.4	37.6	39.3
deeply dark CADBURY	540		7.5	38.4	39.2
Breakaway					
milk chocolate NESTLÉ	500		6.2	61.1	25.6
Buttermints					
BASSETT	405		0.1	91.5	4.3
Caramac					
NESTLÉ	565		5.8	16.3	36
Caramel					
CADBURY	480		4.9	62.3	23.3
GALAXY	482		5	61.3	24
Caramels					
dark chocolate coated	479		3	60.7	25.1
Cherry Drops					
BASSETT	180		0	45.3	0
Chewing Gum					
Airwaves, black mint WRIGLEY	155		0	62	0
Airwaves, cherry menthol WRIGLEY	150		0	62	0

Food Type	cal per 100g	cal per portion	pro (g)	carb (g)	fat (g)
Airwaves, green mint WRIGLEY	156		0	64.7	0
Airwaves, menthol & eucalyptus WRIGLEY	150		0	62	0
Doublemint WRIGLEY	306		0	n/a	0
Extra Cool Breeze WRIGLEY	165		0	64	0
Extra Ice WRIGLEY	147		0	61	0
Extra Peppermint WRIGLEY	155		0	61	0
Extra Spearmint WRIGLEY	158		0	66	0
Orbit, Complete WRIGLEY	150		0	62	0
Orbit, lemon & lime, xylitol WRIGLEY	157		0	63	0
Orbit, peppermint, xylitol WRIGLEY	155		0	60	0
Orbit, spearmint, xylitol WRIGLEY	155		0	60	0
Orbit, strawberry, xylitol WRIGLEY	159		0	60	0
Soft Peppermint TRIDENT	150		0.4	62.3	0.4
Soft Spearmint TRIDENT	155		0.5	63	0.2
Soft Strawberry Smoothie TRIDENT	17		0.5	64.9	0.6
Soft Tropical Twist TRIDENT	155		0.5	60.6	0.6
Spearmint WRIGLEY	281		0	N	0
Splash, apple & apricot TRIDENT	180		1.1	70.4	0.3
Splash, raspberry & peach TRIDENT	180		1.6	68.5	0.5
Splash, strawberry & lime TRIDENT	175		1.6	67.3	0.3
Splash, vanilla & mint TRIDENT	175		1.6	69.8	0.2

Food Type	cal per 100g	cal per portion	pro (g)	carb (g)	fat (g)
Chewits					
chunky chews LEAF	378		0.3	86.9	2.7
extreme apple LEAF	378		0.3	86.9	2.7
strawberry LEAF	378		0.3	86.9	2.7
truly smoothly berry whites LEAF	285		5.1	68	0.2
Chocolate					
milk	520		7.7	56.9	30.7
plain	510		5	63.5	28
white	529		8	58.3	30.9
dark 70%, organic GREEN & BLACK	551		9.3	36	41.1
dark 72% cook's, organic GREEN & BLACK	566		9.6	31.2	44.7
dark 85%, organic GREEN & BLACK	693		9.1	15.7	61.5
milk, organic GREEN & BLACK	523		9.9	54	29.7
white, organic GREEN & BLACK	573		7.4	53.5	36.6
Chocolate Chips, Milk					
fairtrade, organic SUPERCOOK	512		5.8	65.5	26.2
Chocolate Covered Raisins					
JULIAN GRAVES	409		4.2	66.1	14.2
Chocolate Cream, Fry's					
CADBURY	415		2.8	69.9	13.9
Chocolate Drops, Plain					
organic DOVES FARM	505		5.7	58.9	27.4
Chocolate Eclairs					
CADBURY	455		4.5	68.8	17.9

Food Type	cal per 100g	cal per portion	pro (g)	carb (g)	fat (g)
Chocolate Flakes, Milk					
organic DOVES FARM	507		7.8	56.7	27.7
Chocolate Orange					
TERRY'S	530		7.4	58	29.5
Chocolate Orange Segsations					
TERRY'S	525		6.9	58.5	28.5
Chocolate Truffles					
with Amaretto ELIZABETH SHAW	507		4.6	50.5	30.8
with Cointreau ELIZABETH SHAW	526		4.4	54.9	30.9
Chocolate, Almond					
organic GREEN & BLACK	578		11.8	37.7	42.2
Chocolate, Butterscotch					
organic GREEN & BLACK	501		6.8	53	29.1
Chocolate, Cherry					
dark, organic GREEN & BLACK	477		7.9	48	28.2
Chocolate, Dark & Gingerbread					
organic GREEN & BLACK	755		11.4	73.5	46.1
Chocolate, Ginger					
organic GREEN & BLACK	501		6.8	53	29.1
Chocolate, Hazelnut & Currant					
organic GREEN & BLACK	558		8.1	40.3	36.7
Chocolate, Maya Gold					
organic GREEN & BLACK	526		7.3	48.2	33.8
Chocolate, Milk & Spiced Fruit					
organic GREEN & BLACK	744		12	75	43.5

Food Type	cal per 100g	cal per portion	pro (g)	carb (g)	fat (g)
Chocolate, Mint					
organic GREEN & BLACK	478		7.4	50.5	27.3
Chocolate, Raisin & Hazelnut					
organic, each DOVES FARM	556		9.2	46.8	36.9
Chomp					
each CADBURY		110	0.7	16.2	4.8
Cranberry Clusters					
ELIZABETH SHAW	496		6.5	65.6	23
Creme Egg					
each CADBURY		170	1.5	27.7	6
twisted CADBURY		210	2.3	29.1	9.4
Crunch					
milk chocolate NESTLÉ	513		7	62.3	26.2
Crunchie					
CADBURY	500		6.2	64	24.6
Crunchie Nuggets					
CADBURY	470		4.1	71.5	18.8
Curly Wurly					
each CADBURY		115	0.9	18	4.5
Curly Wurly Squirlies					
each CADBURY		205	1.6	31.2	7.9
Dairy Milk Chocolate					
CADBURY	525		7.5	56.7	29.8
99 calories, each CADBURY		95	1.3	9.9	5.3
with creme egg, each CADBURY		210	2.4	29.2	9.4

Food Type	cal per 100g	cal per portion	pro (g)	carb (g)	fat (g)
Dairy Milk Shots					
CADBURY	490		5.7	66.2	22.4
Delight					
MARS	557		4.5	58.9	33.6
Double Choc					
CADBURY	485		6	59.2	24.9
Double Decker					
each CADBURY		275	2.6	41	11.3
Dream					
CADBURY	555		4.5	59.7	33.3
Everton Mints					
BASSETT	395		0.4	93.2	2.1
Flake					
each CADBURY		170	2.6	17.8	9.9
dark, each CADBURY		160	1.8	16.6	9.5
dipped, each CADBURY		210	3	22.4	12.3
praline, each CADBURY		205	3.1	19.3	12.8
Flake Moments					
CADBURY	535		7.6	55	31.7
Freddo					
each CADBURY		105	1.5	11.4	6
Fruit Allsorts					
BASSETT	385		4.5	82.7	3.7
Fruit Gums					
ROWNTREE	332		4.6	78.5	0.2

Food Type	cal per 100g	cal per portion	pro (g)	carb (g)	fat (g)
Fruit Pastilles					
ROWNTREE	351		4.4	84.9	0
Fruit Salad Gums					
JULIAN GRAVES	316		3.3	75.3	0.2
Fruit & Nut Chocolate					
CADBURY	490		8.3	55.8	25.9
Fudge					
each CADBURY		110	0.7	18.4	3.8
Galaxy Chocolate					
MARS	544		6.6	56.3	32.5
fruit & hazelnut MARS	528		6.5	54.7	31.4
hazelnut MARS	568		7.1	49.9	37.7
Glacier					
dark FOX'S CONFECTIONERY	398		2.6	95.1	0.8
fruits FOX'S CONFECTIONERY	387		Tr	96.4	0.1
mints FOX'S CONFECTIONERY	392		0	97.8	Tr
Heaven					
dark truffle NESTLÉ	549		5.3	54.1	38.1
hazelnut creme NESTLÉ	564		6.1	61.8	36.7
milk truffle NESTLÉ	560		5.9	58.1	38
perles caramel latte NESTLÉ	574		6.9	62.5	37.9
perles dark truffle NESTLÉ	569		6.1	57.4	39.2
perles praline NESTLÉ	587		6.2	59.3	40.6
Jelly Babies	334		5.2	78	0
BASSETT	330		3.5	78.9	Tr

Food Type	cal per 100g	cal per portion	pro (g)	carb (g)	fat (g)
milky BASSETT	335		7.2	72.5	1.9
party BASSETT	320		5.3	73.7	0.2
Jellytots					
ROWNTREE	342		0.2	70.9	0
Juicy Jellies					
ROWNTREE	327		4.9	83	0.2
Kinder Bueno					
milk & hazelnut FERRERO	563		9.8	46.6	37.5
Kinder Surprise					
FERRERO	559		9.6	51.7	34.9
Kit Kat					
2-finger cappucino NESTLÉ	510		5.6	10.2	26.7
2-finger mint NESTLÉ	508		6	10.1	26.4
2-finger orange NESTLÉ	507		5.5	10.2	26.5
4-finger dark chocolate NESTLÉ	503		5.4	19.3	28.3
4-finger milk chocolate NESTLÉ	510		5.5	22.8	26.7
chunky milk chocolate NESTLÉ	518		5.2	25.8	28.2
chunky milk chocolate duo					
NESTLÉ	531		5.1	18.8	29.6
chunky peanut butter NESTLÉ	537		8.4	23.9	31.5
chunky peanut butter duo					
NESTLÉ	537		8.4	23.9	31.5
hazelnut senses NESTLÉ	531		7.5	13	30.7
Lion Bar					
NESTLÉ	503		4.8	29	24.9

Food Type	cal per 100g	cal per portion	pro (g)	carb (g)	fat (g)
Liquorice Allsorts					
BASSETT	375		5	79.8	3.9
M & Ms					
chocolate MARS	484		5.1	67.9	21.3
crispy MARS	506		4.4	64.2	25.7
peanut MARS	516		9.8	59	26.8
Maltesers					
MARS	505		7.9	62.8	24.7
Mars Bar					
MARS	448		4.1	68.1	17.6
Matchmakers					
Coolmint NESTLÉ	479		4.1	69.7	20.4
Melts					
deliciously dark CADBURY	575		5.9	47.9	40
heavenly praline CADBURY	560		7.4	49.7	36.9
velvety milk CADBURY	580		6.3	48.7	39.8
Milk Tray					
CADBURY	495		4.7	61.5	25.8
Milky Bar					
NESTLÉ	547		7.3	57.6	31.7
Milky Bar Buttons					
NESTLÉ	547		7.3	57.6	31.7
Milky Way Magic Stars					
MARS	559		6.3	55.3	34.7

Food Type	cal per 100g	cal per portion	pro (g)	carb (g)	fat (g)
Minstrels					
GALAXY	505		5.1	71.6	22
Mint Creams					
BASSETT	365		Tr	91.8	Tr
Mint Crisps					
dark ELIZABETH SHAW	473		2.8	67.4	21.4
milk chocolate ELIZABETH SHAW	499		4.2	68.8	23
orange ELIZABETH SHAW	470		2.8	66.9	21.2
Mint Imperials					
BASSETT	400		0.4	98.1	0.5
Murray Mints					
BASSETT	415		Tr	90.9	5.5
Orange Clusters					
ELIZABETH SHAW	458		5.2	60.7	22.2
Orange Cream, Fry's					
each CADBURY		210	1.4	36.1	7
Pear Drops					
BASSETT	385		Tr	96.4	Tr
Peppermints	393		0.5	102.7	0.7
Peppermint Cream, Fry's					
each CADBURY		215	1.4	36.3	6.8
Picnic					
each CADBURY		225	3.3	27.7	11.1
Planets					
MARS	482		4.8	65.3	22.4

Food Type	cal per 100g	cal per portion	pro (g)	carb (g)	fat (g)
Polo Fruits					
NESTLÉ	387		0	95.7	0
Polo Mints					
NESTLÉ	402		0	98.2	1
spearmint NESTLÉ	401		Tr	98	1
strong NESTLÉ	399		Tr	95.2	1
sugar-free NESTLÉ	238		0	99	0
Poppets					
mint PAYNES	441		1.9	79.4	12.9
raisin PAYNES	401		4.9	65.4	13.3
toffee PAYNES	495		4.4	74.8	19.8
Quality Street					
NESTLÉ	471		4.2	64.6	21.7
Revels					
MARS	481		5.3	66.9	21.3
Ripple					
GALAXY	531		6.7	60.3	29.3
Rolo					
NESTLÉ	471		3.2	69.8	19.9
Roses					
assortment CADBURY	495		4.8	62.6	25.3
luxury assortment CADBURY	550		5.4	54	34.7
truffle selection CADBURY	575		7.6	46	40.4
Sherbert Lemon					
BASSETT	375		Tr	93.3	Tr

Food Type	cal per 100g	cal per portion	pro (g)	carb (g)	fat (g)
Skittles					
MARS	403		0	90.5	4.3
crazy sours MARS	388		87.4	74.6	4.2
Smarties					
NESTLÉ	456		4.2	74.7	17.2
Snack					
sandwich chocolate, each					
CADBURY		135	1.7	15.4	7.4
shortcake, each CADBURY		225	3	27.1	11.4
wafer, each CADBURY		185	2.6	24	9.5
Snakes					
BASSETT	320		3.5	76.8	0.1
Snaps					
CADBURY	505		6.3	60.5	27
caramel crunch CADBURY	510		6.1	59.9	27.6
mint CADBURY	505		6.3	60.2	26.9
orange CADBURY	505		6.3	60.4	27
Snickers					
MARS	511		9.4	54.5	28.4
Softfruits					
per pack (45g) TREBOR		160	0	39.4	0
Softmints					
peppermint TREBOR	355		Tr	88.9	Tr
spearmint, per pack (45g)					
TREBOR		160	0	40	0

Food Type	cal per 100g	cal per portion	pro (g)	carb (g)	fat (g)
Sour Squirms					
BASSETT	325		2.8	78.5	Tr
Spearmint Imperials					
BASSETT	400		0.4	98	0.5
Sports Mix					
MAYNARD'S	345		8.8	46.3	0.2
Starbar					
each CADBURY		275	5.5	28.4	15.3
Starburst					
MARS	403		0	83.4	7.4
choozers MARS	395		0	83.7	6.2
sours MARS	392		0	82	7.1
Sweets					
boiled	327		Tr	87.1	Tr
Sweetshop Favourites					
BASSETT	385		Tr	95.8	Tr
Tasters					
each CADBURY		240	3.4	25.4	13.7
Tic Tac					
lime & orange FERRERO	389		0	96	0
fresh mint FERRERO	390		0	97.5	0
spearmint FERRERO	390		0	97.5	0
Timeout					
each CADBURY		180	2.1	19.8	10.4

Food Type	cal per 100g	cal per portion	pro (g)	carb (g)	fat (g)
Toblerone					
TERRY'S	525		5.4	59	29.5
Toffees					
mixed	426		2.2	66.7	18.6
assorted BASSETT	390		3	63.9	13.3
Toffee Crisp					
NESTLÉ	516		3.7	63.1	27.7
Toffee & Fudge Favourites					
BASSETT	415		1.8	65.2	16.1
Toffo					
NESTLÉ	452		2.1	24.2	18.1
mint NESTLÉ	440		2.2	25.2	15.5
liquorice NESTLÉ	436		2.2	23.8	14.6
Tootie Frooties					
ROWNTREE	397		0.1	91.5	3.5
Topic					
MARS	498		6.2	59.5	26.1
Trebor Extra Cool Mints					
spearmint, per pack TREBOR		65	0	27.2	0
peppermint, per pack TREBOR		65	0	27.2	0
Trebor Extra Strong Mints					
per pack (45g) TREBOR		180	0.01	44.4	0
extra strong spearmint, per pack (45g)		180	0.1	44.4	0

Food Type	cal per 100g	cal per portion	pro (g)	carb (g)	fat (g)
Turkish, Dairy Milk					
CADBURY	465		5.3	63.7	20.8
Turkish Delight, Fry's					
each CADBURY		185	0.8	37.9	3.6
Twirl					
each CADBURY		230	3.2	24.1	13.2
Twix					
MARS	490		4.7	65.5	23.7
Viscount Mint					
BURTON'S	520		5.3	60.1	28.7
Viscount Orange					
BURTON'S	523		5.1	60.1	29.1
Vodka Shots					
all flavours ELIZABETH SHAW	445		3	55.1	20
Walnut Whip					
vanilla NESTLÉ	495		5.9	60.8	25.4
Wholenut Chocolate					
CADBURY	550		8.9	49.5	35.4
Wine Gums					
MAYNARD'S	325		5.8	74.2	0.6
sours MAYNARD'S	330		5.2	75.5	0.5
Wine Pastilles					
MAYNARD'S	330		5.2	76.6	0.5
Wispa					
each CADBURY		210	2.7	21.2	12.9

Food Type	cal per 100g	cal per portion	pro (g)	carb (g)	fat (g)
York Fruits					
TERRY'S	320		Tr	78.5	Tr
Yorkie					
NESTLÉ	537		6.1	60.4	26.8
biscuit NESTLÉ	512		6.3	61.2	26.8
raisin & biscuit NESTLÉ	497		5.5	60.5	26.2

Food Type	cal per 100g	cal per portion	pro (g)	carb (g)	fat (g)
Vegetables					
see also: CONDIMENTS & SAUCES					
Vegetables					
Artichoke, Globe					
base leaves and heart, boiled	18		2.8	2.7	0.2
Artichoke, Jerusalem	77		2	17	0.1
flesh only, boiled	41		1.6	10.6	0.1
Asparagus					
soft tips only, boiled	26		3.4	1.4	0.8
canned, drained	24		3.4	1.5	0.5
green GREEN GIANT	13		1.7	1.7	0.1
white GREEN GIANT	13		0.8	1.8	0.2
Aubergine					
sliced, fried in corn oil	302		1.2	2.8	31.9
Avocado Pear	190		1.9	1.9	19.5
Bamboo Shoots					
sliced, canned	7		0.6	1	0.1
AMOY	22		0.7	3.5	0.2
BLUE DRAGON	17		1.7	2.3	0.2
Beans, Broad					
canned	82		8	11	0.7
frozen, boiled	81		7.9	11.7	0.6
prepack, shelled	77		6	12	0.6
Beans, Green					
trimmed	24		1.9	3.2	0.5

Food Type	cal per 100g	cal per portion	pro (g)	carb (g)	fat (g)
trimmed, boiled	22		1.8	2.9	0.5
canned	24		1.5	3.8	0.3
frozen, whole	25		1.7	4.4	0.1
frozen, sliced	27		1.7	5	0
frozen, boiled	25		1.7	4.7	0.1
canned BONDUELLE	21		1.4	3	0.4
frozen, sliced ROSS	25		1.8	4.4	0.1
Beans, Runner					
trimmed, boiled	18		1.2	2.3	0.5
Beansprouts, Mung	31		2.9	4	0.5
stirfried in blended oil	72		1.9	2.5	6.1
canned BLUE DRAGON	23		1.8	3.4	0.2
Beetroot					
trimmed, peeled	36		1.7	7.6	0.1
trimmed, peeled, boiled	46		2.3	9.5	0.1
pickled, whole & sliced	28		1.2	5.6	0.2
baby BAXTERS	26		1.2	5.1	0.1
baby HAYWARD'S	28		1.1	5.6	0.1
pickled, all varieties BAXTERS	26		1.2	5.1	0.1
Broccoli					
florets, boiled	24		3.1	1.1	0.8
florets, frozen	31		3.3	2.3	0.9
Brussels Sprouts					
trimmed, boiled	35		2.9	3.5	1.3
frozen ROSS	35		3.5	2.4	1.3

Food Type	cal per 100g	cal per portion	pro (g)	carb (g)	fat (g)
Cabbage (January King, Savoy, Summer)					
trimmed	26		1.7	4.1	0.4
boiled in unsalted water	16		1	2.2	0.4
white, trimmed	27		1.4	5	0.2
spring greens	33		3	3.1	1
spring greens, boiled	20		1.9	1.6	0.7
Carrots					
old	35		0.6	7.9	0.3
old, boiled	24		0.6	4.9	0.4
young	30		0.7	6	0.5
young, boiled	22		0.6	4.4	0.3
canned	20		0.5	4.2	0.3
frozen, boiled	22		0.4	4.7	0.3
grated	37		0.6	8	0.3
baby, canned BONDUELLE	19		0.6	3.4	0.3
Carrots, Cauliflower & Green Beans					
Steam Fresh BIRDS EYE	23		1.7	3.6	0.2
Carrots, Sweetcorn & Peas					
Steam Fresh BIRDS EYE	59		3	10.2	0.7
Cassava					
baked	155		0.7	40.1	0.2
boiled	130		0.5	33.5	0.2
fresh	142		0.6	36.8	0.2

Food Type	cal per 100g	cal per portion	pro (g)	carb (g)	fat (g)
Cauliflower	34		3.6	3	0.9
boiled	28		2.9	2.1	0.9
frozen	20		2	1.9	0.5
Cauliflower & Broccoli					
frozen	26		2.7	2.1	0.7
Celeriac					
prepack	29		1.3	5	0.4
flesh only, boiled	15		0.9	1.9	0.5
Celery					
stem only	7		0.5	0.9	0.2
stem only, boiled	8		0.5	0.8	0.3
Chicory	11		0.5	2.8	0.6
Chillies					
whole SCHWARTZ	425		15.9	56.4	15.1
Corn see SWEETCORN					
Courgettes (zucchini)					
trimmed	18		1.8	1.8	0.4
trimmed, boiled	19		2	2	0.4
trimmed, sliced, fried in corn oil	63		2.6	2.6	4.8
Cucumber					
trimmed	10		0.7	1.5	0.1
Fennel, Florence	12		0.9	1.8	0.2
boiled	11		0.9	1.5	0.2
Garlic	98		7.9	16.3	0.6
granules SCHWARTZ	366		15.9	74.6	0.5

Food Type	cal per 100g	cal per portion	pro (g)	carb (g)	fat (g)
minced SCHWARTZ	366		15.9	74.6	0.5
paste ENGLISH PROVENDER	134		4.9	11.3	7.7
sliced, jar ENGLISH PROVENDER	98		98	6.1	16.7
Garlic Purée	423		2.7	13	40
GIA	391		3.3	1.6	41.3
Gherkins					
pickled	14		0.9	2.6	0.1
Ginger, Root	73		1.7	15	0.7
sliced, jar ENGLISH PROVENDER	52		4.3	2.5	2.7
Ginger, Stem					
in syrup BLUE DRAGON	266		0	70	0
Kale, Curly	33		3.4	1.4	1.6
shredded & boiled	24		2.4	1	1.1
Kohlrabi	23		1.6	3.7	0.2
boiled	18		1.2	3.1	0.2
Leeks					
trimmed	22		1.6	2.9	0.5
trimmed, chopped, boiled	21		1.2	2.6	0.7
Lemongrass					
whole, jar BLUE DRAGON	11		0.5	1.9	0.2
Lettuce	14		0.8	1.7	0.5
iceberg	13		0.7	1.9	0.3
mediterranean salad	19		0.9	3.1	0.3
mixed leaf	17		1.1	2.9	0.1
Mange-tout	32		3.6	4.2	0.2

Food Type	cal per 100g	cal per portion	pro (g)	carb (g)	fat (g)
boiled	26		3.2	3.3	0.1
stir-fried	71		3.8	3.5	4.8
Marrow					
flesh only	12		0.5	2.2	0.2
flesh only, boiled	9		0.4	1.6	0.2
Mixed Vegetables					
frozen	39		3.3	4.5	0.9
Mushrooms, Common	13		1.8	0.4	0.5
boiled	11		1.8	0.4	0.3
canned	12		2.1	Tr	0.4
fried in oil	157		2.4	0.3	16.2
Mushrooms, Oyster	8		1.6	0	0.2
Mushrooms, Shiitake					
cooked	55		1.6	12.3	0.2
dried	296		9.6	63.9	1
fresh	8		1.6	0	0.2
Mushrooms, straw					
canned, drained	15		2.1	1.2	0.2
Okra (Gumbo, Lady's Fingers)	31		2.8	3	1
boiled	28		2.5	2.7	0.9
fresh	41		2	8	0.1
stir-fried	269		4.3	4.4	26.1
frozen TAJ	40		2	8	0
Olives					
green, pitted, in brine	103		0.9	Tr	11

Food Type	cal per 100g	cal per portion	pro (g)	carb (g)	fat (g)
black, pitted, in sunflower oil	174		1.1	1.1	18.4
Onions					
flesh only	36		1.2	7.9	0.2
boiled	17		0.6	3.7	0.1
cocktail/silverskin, drained	15		0.6	3.1	0.1
cocktail/silverskin, drained					
HAYWARD'S	10		0.4	1.8	0.1
cocktail/silverskin, drained					
OPIES	36		0.6	8.3	Tr
dried	313		10.2	68.6	1.7
dried WHITWORTHS	331		10.2	68.6	1.7
fried in oil	164		2.3	14.1	11.2
pickled, drained	24		0.9	4.9	0.2
red, caramelised, jar ENGLISH					
PROVENDER	213		1.9	50.9	0.2
Parsnips					
trimmed, peeled, boiled	66		1.6	12.9	1.2
frozen, roasting	139	1.3	20	6	1.2
frozen, roasting, honey glazed					
AUNT BESSIE'S	165	1.3	2.2	14.9	10.7
Peas					
no pod	83		6.9	11.3	1.5
boiled	79		6.7	10	1.6
canned	80		5.3	13.5	0.9
dried, boiled	109		6.9	19.9	0.8

Food Type	cal per 100g	cal per portion	pro (g)	carb (g)	fat (g)
frozen, boiled	69	6	9.7	0.9
Peas, Garden					
frozen	68		5.9	9	0.9
frozen BIRDS EYE	62		4.9	9	0.7
see also: BEANS, PULSES & CEREALS					
see also: PETITS POIS					
Peppers					
green, stalk & seeds removed	15		0.8	2.6	0.3
green, boiled	18		1	2.6	0.5
red, stalk & seeds removed	32		1	6.4	0.4
red, boiled	34		1.1	7	0.4
yellow, stalk & seeds removed	26		1.2	5.3	0.2
mixed, sliced, frozen	28		1.1	4.9	0.4
chilli, green	20		2.9	0.7	0.6
jalapeños, green, sliced					
DISCOVERY FOODS	24		0.8	3.7	0.7
jalapeños, red, sliced					
DISCOVERY FOODS	69		0.4	16.4	0.2
red chilli, jar ENGLISH PROVENDER	52		4.3	2.5	2.7
Petits Pois	100		6.9	17.5	0.8
canned	60		4	11	0
frozen, boiled	49		5	5.5	0.9
frozen	50		5	5.4	0.9
Petits Pois & Baby Carrots					
canned BONDUELLE	45		2.9	7.2	0.5

Food Type	cal per 100g	cal per portion	pro (g)	carb (g)	fat (g)
Petits Pois & Soya Beans					
Steam Fresh BIRDS EYE	90		7.6	9.4	2.4
Pigeon Peas					
frozen, fresh TAJ	301		20	54	2
Potatoes, New					
boiled, peeled	75		1.5	17.8	0.3
boiled in skins	66		1.4	15.4	0.3
canned	63		1.5	15.1	0.1
Potatoes, Old					
baked, flesh & skin	136		3.9	31.7	0.2
baked, flesh only	77		2.2	18	0.1
boiled, peeled	72		1.8	17	0.1
mashed with butter & milk	104		1.8	15.5	4.3
mashed, as prepared AUNT BESSIE'S	115		1.9	14.3	5.1
roast in oil/lard	149		2.9	25.9	4.5
Potato Powder, Instant					
made up with semi-skimmed milk	70		2.4	14.8	1.2
made up with skimmed milk	66		2.4	14.8	0.1
made up with water	57		1.5	13.5	0.1
made up with water SMASH	104		2.5	22.6	0.2
made up with whole milk	76		2.4	14.8	1.2

see also: **CHIPS, FRIES & SHAPED POTATO PRODUCTS**

Food Type	cal per 100g	cal per portion	pro (g)	carb (g)	fat (g)
Pumpkin					
flesh only	13		0.7	2.2	0.2
flesh only, boiled	13		0.6	2.1	0.3
Raddiccio	14		1.4	1.7	0.2
Radish, Red	12		0.7	1.9	0.2
Radish, White (Mooli)	15		0.8	2.9	0.1
Ratatouille					
canned	50		1	7	2
Roast Mix					
as prepared AUNT BESSIE'S	301		4.8	41.9	12.7
Salsify					
flesh only	27		1.3	10.2	0.3
flesh only, boiled	23		1.1	8.6	0.4
Shallots	20		1.5	3.3	0.2
boiled	19		2.2	0.8	0.8
Spinach	25		2.8	1.6	0.8
frozen, boiled	21		3.1	0.5	0.8
Spring Onions, Bulbs & Tops	23		2	3	0.5
Stir Fry Vegetables					
AMOY	139		4.9	28.8	1.1
canned BLUE DRAGON	26		1.1	3.1	1
Sushi Nori					
BLUE DRAGON	455		45.5	91	0
Swede					
flesh only, boiled	11		0.3	2.3	0.1

Food Type	cal per 100g	cal per portion	pro (g)	carb (g)	fat (g)
Sweet Potato					
boiled	84		1.1	20.5	0.3
with rosemary & garlic, as					
prepared MCCAIN	115		2.1	18.4	3.7
Sweetcorn					
on cob	110		4.2	18	2.3
mini corncobs, canned	23		2.9	2	0.4
mini corncobs, fresh/frozen,					
boiled	24		2.5	2.7	0.4
giant baby cobs GREEN GIANT	28		1.8	4.7	0.3
Sweetcorn, Kernels					
canned, drained, re-heated	122		2.9	26.6	1.2
frozen BIRDS EYE	93		2.9	18.4	0.9
Niblets, canned GREEN GIANT	100		2.7	20.8	0.7
Niblets, naturally sweet GREEN					
GIANT	77		2.6	16.7	0
Niblets, Salad Crisp GREEN GIANT	70		2.7	13.3	0.7
Niblets, with peppers GREEN GIANT	82		2.6	17.9	0
Tindora (Indian Gourd)					
frozen TAJ	22		2.5	3	0
Tomatoes	19		0.7	3.1	0.4
canned, whole	16		1	3	0.1
cherry	18		0.7	3.1	0.3
fried in oil!	91		0.7	5	7.7

Food Type	cal per 100g	cal per portion	pro (g)	carb (g)	fat (g)
grilled	20		0.8	3.5	0.3
sun-dried	209		4.3	11	16.4
Tomatoes, Chopped, Canned					
NAPOLINA	22		1.1	3.5	0.4
cherry NAPOLINA	23		1.2	3.3	0.6
organic NAPOLINA	22		1.1	3.5	0.4
with garlic NAPOLINA	24		1.3	4.3	0.2
with herbs NAPOLINA	24		1.3	4.3	0.2
Tomatoes, Sieved					
passata	25		1.4	4.5	0.1
passata NAPOLINA	25		1.4	4.5	0.1
passata, organic MERIDIAN FOODS	28		1.2	4.8	0.5
Tomato Purée					
purée	76		5	14.2	0.3
HEINZ	57		3.7	10.1	0.2
NAPOLINA	73		4.7	12.6	0.4
sun-dried GIA	204		2.6	Tr	21.6
Turnips					
flesh only	23		0.9	4.7	0.3
flesh only, boiled	12		0.6	2	0.2
Water Chestnuts					
canned	28		1.7	4.7	0.3
canned AMOY	25		1.8	3.7	0.3
canned BLUE DRAGON	35		0.9	8.5	0

Food Type	cal per 100g	cal per portion	pro (g)	carb (g)	fat (g)
Yam					
flesh only	114		1.5	28.2	0.3
flesh only, boiled	133		1.7	33	0.3
Chips, Fries and Shaped Potato Products					
Non-branded Chips					
crinkle cut, frozen, for frying	168		2.3	24	7
crinkle cut, frozen, oven baking	134		2	23	3.8
French fries, retail	280		3.3	34	15.5
homemade, fried	189		3.9	30.1	6.7
microwave	221		3.6	32.1	9.6
oven	162		3.2	29.8	4.2
retail	239		3.2	30.5	12.4
straight cut, frozen, fried	273		4.1	36	13.5
Beer Battered Chips					
as prepared MCCAIN	220		2.3	29.7	10.1
Chippy Chips					
as prepared MCCAIN	176		2.5	26.8	6.5
Chips					
crinkle cut, as prepared AUNT BESSIE'S	206		2.9	28	9.2
Chunky, Simply Gorgeous, as prepared MCCAIN	253		2.3	24	16.4
Homestyle, as prepared AUNT BESSIE'S	191		3.1	27	7.8

Food Type	cal per 100g	cal per portion	pro (g)	carb (g)	fat (g)
Crispy Bites					
as prepared MCCAIN	187		3.4	27.8	5.4
Crispy Slices					
as prepared MCCAIN	240		3.2	32.1	8.5
Croquettes					
potato, fried in oil	214		3.7	21.6	13.1
chunky, as prepared AUNT BESSIE'S	170		3.3	23.1	7.2
chunky, as prepared MCCAIN	168		3	22.7	7.2
Curly Fries					
as prepared MCCAIN	195		2.1	23.7	10.2
French Fries					
as prepared MCCAIN	193		1.9	27.4	8.5
crispy, as prepared MCCAIN	270		4.3	38.8	10.9
Hash Browns					
as prepared MCCAIN	191		1.5	31.4	7.6
Home Fries					
as prepared MCCAIN	181		3.1	28.1	6.2
chunky, as prepared MCCAIN	153		3.2	28	3.1
crinkle cut, as prepared MCCAIN	197		3	31.7	6.5
thin & crispy, as prepared MCCAIN	225		4	36.9	6.8
Micro Chips					
MCCAIN	163		2.3	27.7	4.8
crinkle cut, as prepared MCCAIN	166		2.9	28.9	4.2

Vegetables

Food Type	cal per 100g	cal per portion	pro (g)	carb (g)	fat (g)
Oven Chips					
crinkle cut, as prepared MCCAIN	163		3.1	27.9	4.3
rustic, as prepared AUNT BESSIE'S	149		2.8	24	4.7
rustic, as prepared MCCAIN	136		3.4	25.5	2.3
straight cut, as prepared MCCAIN	172		3.4	32.4	4.9
Potato Gourmet					
cheddar & wholegrain mustard gratin, as prepared MCCAIN	150		3.6	16.5	7.8
diced potatoes with leeks, onions & parmesan, as prepared MCCAIN	166		3.2	19.2	8.5
spicy potato bravas, as prepared MCCAIN	100		1.7	17.6	2.6
Potato Waffles					
frozen, as sold BIRDS EYE	175		2.5	21.6	8.7
frozen, cooked ROSS	225		2.3	22	12.3
Roast Potatoes					
crispy, as prepared AUNT BESSIE'S	178		2.5	24.2	8
home, as prepared MCCAIN	147		2.9	26	3.5
rustic, as prepared MCCAIN	117		2	23.9	1.6
Rosti					
as prepared MCCAIN	194		2.6	25	9.3
Smiles					
as prepared MCCAIN	237		3.4	33.4	10.1

Food Type	cal per 100g	cal per portion	pro (g)	carb (g)	fat (g)
Southern Fries					
as prepared MCCAIN	228		3.4	34.7	8.5
Wedges, Oven Baked					
MCCAIN	173		3.3	30.2	4.3
lightly spiced MCCAIN	187		2.8	26.5	7.7
mexican chilli MCCAIN	230		5.2	37.2	8.8
ridge cut MCCAIN	168		2.1	25.2	6.5
sea salt & black pepper MCCAIN	175		3.1	26.6	6.2
winter herb MCCAIN	181		2.3	28.4	6.4
Vegetable Roasties					
LINDA MCCARTNEY FOODS	151		4.7	19	6.2

Vegetables

Recipes

Most of the recipes serve four; any exceptions
are clearly indicated. Recipes that are adapted
to serve a different number of people may
require adjustments to cooking times, so be aware
of this. All ovens are different, too, so you may
need to make adjustments there as well; the
temperatures given are for a conventional, not fan,
oven. The calorie values are generally approximate
(not all 'medium' onions weigh exactly the same,
for instance) but are accurate enough, and
do not include any suggested accompaniments
or optional additions.

Quick hummus

1 x 400g tin chickpeas
2 cloves of garlic
juice of 1 lemon
2 tbsp tahini

Drain and rinse the chickpeas. Put them in a pan
with fresh water and heat gently for 4 minutes.

Drain, reserving some of the liquid. Crush the garlic, then put the chickpeas in a food processor with the garlic and lemon juice. Add the tahini and a tablespoon of the cooking liquid and process until smooth, adding more liquid if necessary. Serve with pitta chips (see below) and strips of raw vegetables.

Calories: about 125 per portion

Yoghurt and feta cheese dip

200g feta cheese
200g low- or no-fat Greek yoghurt
1 tsp olive oil
a handful of mint

Drain and rinse the feta cheese, then break it up in a bowl using a fork. Add the yoghurt and mix the two together well, beating the yoghurt in and breaking up the cheese further. Finely chop most of the mint, then add the oil and the chopped mint to the yoghurt and mix once more. Garnish with the remaining mint and serve with pitta chips and crudités.

Calories: 170 per portion

Tzatsiki

 1 medium cucumber
 2 cloves of garlic
 a handful of flat-leaved parsley or coriander
 a few mint leaves
 200ml low-fat Greek yoghurt
 ½ tsp olive oil
 cayenne and black pepper

Cut the cucumber in half across, then cut each part in half lengthwise. Remove the seeds and chop the cucumber finely. Chop the herbs, put them in a bowl and add the cucumber; crush the garlic into the bowl as well and stir everything together. Add the yoghurt and mix well. Drizzle the olive oil on top and sprinkle with cayenne and some freshly ground black pepper. Serve with crudités and pitta chips.

Calories: about 50 per portion

Pitta chips

 4 wholemeal pitta breads

Preheat the oven to 160°C/gas mark 2. Cut the pittas in half across and then cut each section into half. Separate the tops and bottoms of each piece and spread them on a baking sheet in a single layer. Bake for about 10 minutes until dry and crispy – but not burned.

Calories: about 135 per portion

Red pepper and tomato soup

Recipes

2 red peppers
2 cloves of garlic
1 medium onion
1 tsp olive oil
1 x 400g tin of tomatoes
75g potatoes
water

Halve the peppers, deseed them and chop them into chunks; chop the onion and garlic. Pour the oil into a heavy-bottomed pan over a medium heat and allow it to warm. Then add the peppers, onion and garlic and allow them to soften for 5 minutes, stirring to make sure they don't stick. Add the tinned tomatoes and potatoes and enough water to cover; if you use the empty tomato tin to measure the water you get all the juice and will need about two refills. Simmer the soup for about 20 minutes until the vegetables are done, then allow them to cool slightly and blend until smooth. Reheat and serve.

Calories: about 70 per portion

Spiced squash soup

1 tsp olive oil
1 small onion
1 clove of garlic
half a butternut squash – about 250g
1 litre vegetable stock or water
1 pinch cayenne pepper

Heat the oil in a large pan. Peel and chop the onion and garlic and add them to the pan and cook gently for 5 minutes; don't allow them to burn. While they are cooking, prepare the squash: cut it into sections, remove the seeds and cut away the peel, then cut any large pieces into smaller chunks. Add the squash to the pan and stir well, then add the stock and a pinch of cayenne. Cook for 20 minutes; allow to cool slightly and then blend. You can adjust the thickness at this point by adding a little more liquid if necessary. Reheat and serve.

Calories: 150 per portion

Onion soup

    800g white onions
    2 cloves of garlic
    10g unsalted butter
    2 tsp olive oil
    500ml dry cider

Slice some of the onions into rings, and chop the rest; chop the garlic finely. Melt the butter with the oil in a large lidded pan over a very gentle heat. Add the onions and garlic and stir well, then allow them to cook slowly over the same gentle heat for about 45 minutes. Do not let them brown (putting the lid on the pan will help). When the onion is soft, transparent and sweet, and much reduced in bulk, add the cider and the same quantity of water – use the cider bottle as a measure. Cook with the lid off for another 10–15 minutes and serve; you can add a little grated cheddar if you wish. This soup is also good the following day.

Calories: 185 per portion

Chunky leek and potato soup

1kg leeks, untrimmed
400g potatoes
2 tsp olive oil
a sprig of fresh thyme
200ml skimmed milk

Trim the leeks, cut them into slices, rinse to dislodge any soil and put them into cold water. Cut the potatoes into 2-cm cubes (leave the skin on). Put the oil in a large pan over a medium heat. Drain the leeks and add them to the pan once the oil has warmed. Cook gently for about 5 minutes; don't allow them to brown. Add the potatoes and the leaves from the thyme, and enough water to cover. Cover the pan with a lid and cook the vegetables for 15–20 minutes, then add the milk and cook for another 20 minutes, adjusting the level of liquid by adding more water if necessary. By now some of the potatoes should be falling apart; if not, break some up with a fork. Test for seasoning and serve.

Calories: about 150 per portion

Lentil and spinach soup

- 100g green lentils
- 1 medium onion
- large clove of garlic
- 1 tsp olive oil
- 175–200g fresh spinach (or kale or spring greens), washed and chopped
- 800ml vegetable stock or water

Check the lentils for the presence of any small stones, then rinse them under running water. Cook them in fresh water for 10–15 minutes, by which time they should be beginning to soften; drain and rinse them again. Peel and chop the onion and garlic. Put the oil in a large pan and cook the onion, allowing it to soften but not burn, then add the garlic and lentils. Wash and chop the spinach and add it to the pan gradually, allowing it to shrink down, and keep stirring. When all the spinach is in, and reduced in bulk by about half, add enough liquid to cover and cook for about 10 minutes – a comparatively short cooking time will maintain the colour of the spinach. Allow to cool slightly, blend, reheat and serve.

Calories: just over 110 per portion

Tomato and feta cheese salad

6–8 large ripe tomatoes
half a small red onion
16 olives
125g feta cheese
2 tsp olive oil
1 tsp balsamic vinegar or lemon juice

Cut the tomatoes into fat slices and layer them on a large plate. Slice the onion into fine rings and scatter them over the tomatoes, then chop the olives and add them too. Drain and rinse the feta and crumble it over the tomatoes, and drizzle the oil and balsamic vinegar over everything.

Calories: 140–150 per portion

Potato salad

500g small or new potatoes
1 tbsp low-fat mayonnaise
3 tbsp low-fat Greek yoghurt
1 tsp Dijon mustard
6 spring onions
half a cucumber

Bring a large pan of water to the boil. Don't peel the potatoes; just chop them into chunks about

2-cm square. Put the potatoes into the water and cook for 15–20 minutes or until tender. While they're cooking, make the dressing: mix the low-fat mayonnaise and yoghurt together, then add the mustard and mix it in well. Drain the potatoes and put them in a large bowl. Allow them to cool a little and then add the dressing; stir them together carefully. Put the salad aside to cool down. Chop the spring onions and cucumber, and add them to the salad once the potatoes are cold; mix well, check the seasoning and serve.

Calories: about 120 per person

Tuna and cannellini bean salad

> 1 x 410g tin of cannellini beans
> 12 sun-dried tomatoes in oil
> 1 medium red onion
> 1 x 185g tin of tuna in brine or spring water
> 1–2 tbsp balsamic vinegar
> juice of half a lemon

Drain and rinse the cannellini beans and put them in a pan with enough water to cover them. Warm them over a gentle heat for 4–5 minutes. Meanwhile, blot the sun-dried tomatoes of excess oil using kitchen roll and cut them into strips; put them in a large bowl. Peel and chop the onion and add that to the bowl as well. Drain the tuna – and rinse it too, if in brine – and flake it into the bowl. Remove the beans from the heat, drain them well, and add them to the bowl. Mix everything together, then add the balsamic vinegar and lemon juice, stir and allow the beans to cool before serving the salad on a bed of lettuce.

Calories: about 135 per portion

Mushroom and garlic pâté

250g mushrooms
2 fat cloves of garlic
a sprig of fresh thyme
15g butter
lots of black pepper
250g carton of extra low-fat soft cheese

Wipe the mushrooms and chop them finely; chop the garlic and strip the leaves from the thyme sprig. Melt the butter in a large frying pan and add the mushrooms, garlic and thyme. Cook, stirring frequently, until all the liquid shed by the cooking mushrooms has evaporated; this should take about 10 minutes. Add the black pepper and allow the mushrooms to cool for 5 minutes, then put them in a food processor and whizz until quite smooth. Add the cheese and process again until well mixed. Test the seasoning and adjust if necessary. Spoon the mixture into a serving dish, cover and refrigerate for at least an hour before serving.

Calories: 117 per portion

Cheddar and chive omelette (serves 1)

25g strong cheddar cheese
a few chives
2 medium eggs
salt and black pepper
10g butter

Grate the cheese and chop the chives. Beat the eggs in a bowl with a teaspoon of water, some salt and black pepper. Add most of the grated cheese and the chives to the egg mixture and beat again. Put a sliver of butter (no more than 10g, though you could use less) in a non-stick omelette or small frying pan. When it begins to froth slightly, pour the eggs into the pan. Swirl them around, leave them alone for a few seconds and then stir them gently, drawing the cooking mix in from the sides towards the middle, and tilt the pan, letting any uncooked liquid run to the edges. Stop stirring when the eggs are really beginning to set and cook for about a minute more. Then fold the omelette in half in the pan and slide it onto a plate. Scatter the remaining cheese on top and serve with a green salad.

Calories: 350

Pasta with cherry tomatoes

400g cherry tomatoes
24 black olives
1 clove of garlic, peeled
a handful of basil
2 tsp olive oil
400g wholewheat pasta
salt and black pepper

Chop the tomatoes, olives and garlic (using as much of the latter as you like). Put them into a bowl with some basil, then drizzle with the oil and stir well. Put the bowl to one side while you cook the pasta in some boiling water. Once the pasta is ready, drain it, rinse with boiling water and return to the pan. Add the tomato mixture and stir thoroughly over a low heat (gas) or on a cooling electric ring. Add some salt and lots of black pepper, and serve immediately.

Calories: about 420 per portion

Pasta with peppers

4 peppers (different colours)
1 medium red onion
1 clove of garlic
2 tsp oil
400g wholewheat penne
salt and black pepper

Halve the peppers and remove the seeds and membranes. Rub the skins with a little olive oil and place them, skin sides up, on a piece of foil under a hot grill. The skins will blister and brown. When this has happened, remove the peppers from the grill, allow them to cool slightly and pull the skin off (it is sometimes easier if you pop them in a plastic bag for a moment). Then slice the peppers and put them into a bowl. Chop the onion and garlic. Put the pasta in a pan of boiling water and cook it. While the pasta is cooking, put 2 tsp oil in a large frying pan and gently fry the onion and garlic. Add the peppers and their juices from the bowl and continue cooking, stirring them together; add a couple of spoonfuls of pasta liquid to keep the sauce moist if necessary. When the pasta is ready, drain and return it to the pan. Add the pepper sauce, salt and lots of black pepper. Stir thoroughly and serve.

Calories: 430 per portion

Steak with mustard sauce and baked potato chips

    4 fillet steaks, about 150g each
    50ml red wine
    100ml low-fat Greek yoghurt
    4 tsp Dijon mustard
    a handful of fresh thyme
    2 tsp olive oil

For the chips:
4 medium baking potatoes, about 175g each
2 tsp olive oil

Trim any excess fat from the steaks and put them in a glass or china dish. Pour the wine into the dish and turn the steaks over in it; cover and set to one side for an hour.

About 30 minutes before you want to serve the steaks, prepare the potatoes. Preheat the oven to 200°C/gas mark 6. Wash the potatoes and then, leaving the peel on, slice them into fat chips. Put them in a pan of water, bring to the boil and cook for 2 minutes. Pour the olive oil into a large roasting dish and pop it into the oven to warm. Drain the potatoes and put them into the dish, and bake for 20–25 minutes, until they are browning nicely, turning them halfway through. Just before you are ready to cook the steaks, make the sauce by mixing the yoghurt, mustard and thyme leaves together thoroughly; once mixed, put in a serving bowl. Heat a large frying pan or ridged griddle with 2 tsp oil. When this is really hot – and starting to smoke – add the steaks and cook to taste, turning them over. Serve them immediately, accompanied by the sauce, potatoes and a green salad.

Calories: steaks, about 250 each; sauce 40 per person; potatoes around 155 per person

Mild chicken curry with lemon and coconut

4 skinless chicken breasts, 125–150g each
1 large onion
1 clove of garlic
4 tsp vegetable oil
2 cm piece of fresh ginger
½ tsp garam masala
½ tsp turmeric
¼ tsp cayenne pepper
juice of 1 lemon
1 tbsp tomato purée
300ml water or vegetable stock
1 tbsp desiccated coconut

Cut the chicken breasts into cubes and finely chop the onion and garlic. Put 2 tsp oil into a large, heavy pan over a medium heat; add the chicken pieces after a minute or so and cook them, stirring, to seal. Once they have coloured slightly, remove them from the pan, add another 2 tsp oil, the onions and garlic. Cook for 2–3 minutes, then grate in the ginger and add the spices. Stir them around, then return the chicken pieces to the pan and add the lemon juice, tomato purée and water. Bring the curry to the boil, then reduce the heat and simmer, stirring occasionally, for 15 minutes. Now add the coconut and top up the level of liquid if necessary – this isn't a wet curry, but it shouldn't be very dry either. Cook for 15 more minutes, covered, until the chicken is tender. Serve with boiled basmati rice.

Calories: 225–255 per portion

Mushroom risotto

2 medium onions
1 clove of garlic
500g mushrooms
2 tsp olive oil
320g risotto rice
about 1 litre boiling water
40g Parmesan cheese, grated
a bunch of parsley, chopped
salt and black pepper

Chop the onions and garlic, and wipe over the mushrooms before chopping them, too. Warm the oil in a large pan; add the onions and garlic and cook gently for 2 minutes. Then add the mushrooms and cook for another minute or so. Add the risotto rice and stir well to coat the rice. After another minute, add enough of the hot liquid to cover the rice and cook, stirring, until the liquid has been absorbed. Then add more liquid, and allow it to be absorbed too (you can also use vegetable stock, but keep it hot). Repeat this process, stirring as you do, until the rice is ready – there should be a bit of 'bite', but it should not be hard – and then take the pan off the heat. Stir in the Parmesan and chopped parsley, check the seasoning and serve.

Calories: about 365 per person

Sea bass parcels

8 sun-dried tomatoes in oil
1 small red onion
4 sea bass fillets, about 175–200g each
juice of 1 lemon

Preheat the oven to 200°C/gas mark 6. Drain the oil from the sun-dried tomatoes and then blot them on several layers of kitchen roll; chop into pieces. Cut the onion into rings. Use four pieces of kitchen foil, each large enough to wrap a piece of fish, and place a fillet on each one. Then scatter the onion rings and sun-dried tomatoes on the sea bass, and pour a little lemon juice over them. Bring the foil up around the sides and fold it into a loose parcel over the top, wrapping the edges together to seal the parcels. Put the foil parcels in a large ovenproof dish, and bake for 20 minutes (check after 12–15 minutes if your fillets are small in size). Serve with a green salad.

Calories: about 225–250 per portion, depending on the size of fish fillets

Roast winter vegetable couscous

2 medium onions
2 medium parsnips
4 medium carrots
2 cloves of garlic
1 x 400g tin of chickpeas
2 tsp olive oil
1 medium butternut squash
pinch of cinnamon
juice of a lemon
200ml water
160g couscous
a handful of fresh coriander leaves

Preheat the oven to 200°C/gas mark 6. Peel and chop the onions, parsnips, carrots and garlic; drain and rinse the chickpeas and set them to one side. Put the oil in a large roasting dish and place it in the oven to warm. Add the chopped vegetables, stir to coat them in the oil and spread them out. Bake for 5 minutes. While they are cooking, chop, deseed and peel the squash, cutting it into 2-cm chunks. Then add those to the roasting tin, together with the cinnamon and lemon juice, and mix well. Roast for a further 15 minutes and then add the drained chickpeas and the water. Continue cooking for a further 10 minutes. Meanwhile, make the couscous according to the instructions on the packet. Put a portion of couscous on each plate, surround with the roasted vegetables and serve, garnished with the coriander and accompanied with some harissa and a green salad.

If the vegetables look a bit dry, add 100ml water to the empty roasting tin after removing them, swirl it around and allow the heat to warm it up, then strain the liquid into a small jug and pour it over the couscous.

Calories: about 250 per portion

Chicken with rosemary and lemon

juice of 1 lemon
a large sprig of rosemary
2 tsp olive oil
4 skinless chicken breasts, 125–150g each
100ml dry white wine

Preheat the oven to 200°C/gas mark 6. Mix the lemon juice, rosemary and olive oil together in a bowl and roll the chicken breasts in it, one by one. Put them in a large glass or china ovenproof dish in a single layer, then add the wine and any remaining lemon juice and rosemary mixture. Cover the dish with foil and bake the chicken for 15 minutes. Remove the foil and cook for another 15 minutes, or until the chicken is done.

Calories: 175–205 per portion

Lamb kebabs

    750g lean lamb steaks
    100g low-fat yoghurt
    1 tsp olive oil
    2 medium onions
    several fresh sprigs of rosemary

Cut the lamb into 2-cm cubes, removing any extra fat. Put the cubes into a large bowl, pour the yoghurt over them and add the olive oil. Turn the lamb over in the yoghurt thoroughly, ensuring all the pieces are slightly coated, and cover the bowl. Chill for at least 4 hours; overnight is best. The next day, take the lamb out of the fridge and cut the onions into chunks.

Thread the onion and lamb onto skewers (if using bamboo skewers, soak them first). Cook them over a hot barbecue or under a pre-heated grill, lying them on the fresh sprigs of rosemary, until they are done to your taste. Serve with a salad made with crunchy lettuce; tzatsiki would be a good low-calorie accompaniment.

Calories: approximately 325 per portion.

Poached salmon

4 salmon fillets, about 130g each
1 lemon
1 bay leaf
a sprig of thyme
half a small onion
water

Preheat the oven to 190° C/gas mark 5. Put the salmon fillets in an ovenproof dish. Cut the lemon in half and squeeze the halves over the fish, then put the squeezed pieces in the dish, too. Add the bay leaf and the spring of thyme. Chop the onion roughly and add that as well. Now add enough water to come halfway up the side of the fish and cover the dish well with foil. Put it in the oven and cook the salmon for 10 minutes. Check the fish and, if further cooking is needed – it should be opaque – take the foil off and cook for another 5 minutes. Remove the dish from the oven and lift the fillets out carefully using a fish slice. They can be served immediately but are delicious cold, perhaps accompanied by potato salad.

Calories: about 235 per fillet

Baked apples with lime

8 small dessert apples, such as Cox
juice of 2 limes
4 tsp brown sugar

Preheat the oven to 180° C/gas mark 4. Quarter the apples and slice them into thinner segments, but leave the peel on. Lightly butter 4 ramekins using the wrapper from a pack of butter. Cram the apple slices into each dish, pressing them down. Sprinkle the lime juice and then the sugar over the apple slices and bake for 20–25 minutes until the tops are browned nicely. Serve with some no- or low-fat Greek yoghurt.

Calories: about 77 per portion

Poached plums with honey

4 plums
2 tsp honey
200ml water

Halve the plums, removing the stones, and put the halves in a large pan. Add the honey and water, and bring the pan to a simmer. Cook for about 10–15 minutes; the plums should not disintegrate completely but retain some bite. Remove them from the pan using a slotted spoon and put them into serving bowls. Increase the temperature and boil the liquid, stirring, until the sauce has reduced by half. Pour it over the plums, and allow to cool slightly before serving.

Calories: about 100 per portion

Highland brose

4 tbsp oatmeal
15g chopped almonds
300g low- or no-fat Greek yoghurt
100g low-fat crème fraîche
8 dried apricots, chopped finely (unsulphured if possible)
1 tbsp whisky
1 tbsp heather honey

Put the oatmeal and chopped almonds on a baking tray and spread them out. Place the tray under a hot grill until they begin to smell warm and toasted; stir them around and give them a few more minutes – they should be golden, not burned. Pour them onto a plate and allow to cool. Mix the yoghurt and crème fraîche together and add the oatmeal and almond mix; stir well and add the apricots, whisky and honey and stir again. Decant the mixture into serving glasses – it's quite rich, so you don't need a large quantity – and chill in the fridge for an hour before serving.

Calories: 176 per portion

Red and black fruit salad

200g watermelon
200g black grapes
1 tbsp Grand Marnier
squeeze of lemon juice
100g ripe strawberries

Cut the skin from the watermelon flesh and remove as many seeds as you can. Then cut the watermelon into pieces, removing any more seeds, and halve the grapes. Put them in a bowl with the Grand Marnier and lemon juice, cover and chill for an hour. Cut the strawberries into pieces and stir them in, too, just before serving.

Calories: 65 per portion

Nectarines in orange juice

6 large nectarines
juice of 3–4 medium oranges
8 amaretti biscuits

Preheat the oven to 180° C/gas mark 4. Cut the nectarines into quarters, removing their stones. Place them in an ovenproof dish, skin side up. Pour the orange juice over them and bake for 20 minutes. Allow them to cool slightly before serving and divide into portions; serve each one accompanied by two amaretti. They are also very good cold, served with some Greek yoghurt or low-fat crème fraîche.

Calories: 145 per portion, including the amaretti

Raspberry and vanilla granita

225g raspberries
75g vanilla sugar
300ml water

Put all the ingredients in a pan and cook them
gently until the sugar has dissolved and the
raspberries have broken up. Put a sieve over a
large bowl and gradually decant the liquid into it;
help the juices through with a wooden spoon but
don't squeeze too hard – you want the juice, not
a purée. Allow the liquid to cool for an hour and
leave the sieve over the bowl to continue
dripping. Pour the liquid into a freezer container
and freeze for 1–2 hours, then remove the
container from the freezer and mash up the
partly frozen contents thoroughly, using a fork.
Return to the freezer and repeat after another 2
hours; you will end up with crystals of deep pink
raspberry ice with an intense flavour.

Calories: 90 per portion

INDEX

Food Diary

Monday

Breakfast:

Lunch:

Dinner:

Anytime:

Food Diary

Tuesday

Breakfast:

Lunch:

Dinner:

Anytime:

Food Diary

Breakfast:

Lunch:

Dinner:

Anytime:

Food Diary

Thursday

Breakfast:

Lunch:

Dinner:

Anytime:

Food Diary

Friday

Breakfast:

Lunch:

Dinner:

Anytime:

Food Diary

Saturday

Breakfast:

Lunch:

Dinner:

Anytime:

Food Diary

Sunday

Breakfast:

Lunch:

Dinner:

Anytime: